T0309255

Understanding
Diabetic
Foot

A Comprehensive
Guide for General
Practitioners

Understanding
Diabetic
Foot

A Comprehensive Guide for General Practitioners

Edited by

Aziz Nather

Consultant Orthopaedic & Diabetic Foot Surgeon
National University Health Services, Singapore

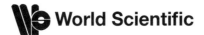

NEW JERSEY · LONDON · SINGAPORE · BEIJING · SHANGHAI · HONG KONG · TAIPEI · CHENNAI · TOKYO

Published by

World Scientific Publishing Co. Pte. Ltd.

5 Toh Tuck Link, Singapore 596224

USA office: 27 Warren Street, Suite 401-402, Hackensack, NJ 07601

UK office: 57 Shelton Street, Covent Garden, London WC2H 9HE

Library of Congress Control Number: 2023000327

British Library Cataloguing-in-Publication Data
A catalogue record for this book is available from the British Library.

UNDERSTANDING DIABETIC FOOT
A Comprehensive Guide for General Practitioners

ISBN 978-981-126-935-6 (hardcover)
ISBN 978-981-126-936-3 (ebook for institutions)
ISBN 978-981-126-937-0 (ebook for individuals)

For any available supplementary material, please visit
https://www.worldscientific.com/worldscibooks/10.1142/13235#t=suppl

Desk Editors: Aanand Jayaraman/Joy Quek

Typeset by Stallion Press
Email: enquiries@stallionpress.com

Foreword

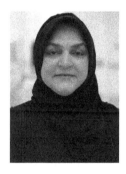

I first met Prof. Aziz Nather in Malaysia in 2019 at the 19th Asia Pacific Diabetic Limb Conference and found him to be a very enthusiastic and passionate writer especially focusing on diabetic foot problems and eager to teach doctors and nurses what to do and how to save limbs.

Associate Prof. Aziz Nather is a Senior Consultant Orthopaedic Surgeon, Visiting Consultant to the Department of Orthopaedic Surgery at Jurong Medical Centre, National University Health Services, Singapore.

As you all know, early identification of high-risk foot and prompt management may save lives, save limbs, and prevent foot ulcers that could result in a better quality of life. Patients with diabetes are at high risk for foot ulceration and lower extremity amputations. Diabetic foot ulcer has one of the most expensive treatments but also one of the most preventable problems through daily foot exam. Successful diagnosis and treatment of patients with diabetic foot ulcers involve a holistic approach. I am so happy to share with you that these are all covered in his book *Understanding Diabetic Foot: A Comprehensive Guide for General Practitioners*.

It is written as a practical guide for general practitioners who commonly treat such patients. Topics covered in this book include the pathogenesis of diabetic foot, the types of diabetic foot complications, the anatomy and biomechanics of the foot, and how to examine and how to treat diabetic foot. The latter includes how to choose the appropriate dressing and the appropriate antibiotic.

A chapter especially useful to GPs is a practical guide on when they are advised to refer their patients to specialists in hospitals. The book also contains a section on patient education: care of diabetes, care of the foot, and choice of footwear. This will be very useful to assist GPs to educate their patients on how to better take care of their diabetes and diabetic foot complications.

While the book has been written specially to meet the needs of GPs, other professionals such as nurses and podiatrists will also find this book to be a useful reading material. To value-add information relevant to the latter professionals, Dr. Nather has added a supplement. Topics include team approach, types of dressings, negative pressure wound therapy, maggot debridement therapy, offloading diabetic foot, and hyperbaric oxygen therapy.

This textbook is a useful practical guide not only to GPs but also to all doctors, medical students, nurses, podiatrists, and other allied health professionals in the ASEAN and Asia Pacific region. It will also benefit professionals practising in other regions including Europe, Central Asia, Australia, and Latin America.

It is my absolute pleasure to write a foreword for such a book which will improve the quality of life for patients with diabetic foot problems.

Gulnaz Tariq
RN, RM, POST GRAD (PAK) IIWCC (Tehran, By UOT) MSc (UK)
President, World Union of Wound Healing Society
CEO, International Interprofessional Wound Care Group (IIWCG)
Clinical Advisor Debra Pakistan
Member of ISWCAP
E-Mail: Gulnaz.t5@gmail.com

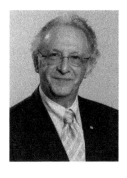

It is with great pleasure that I write the foreword to this new book on *Understanding Diabetic Foot: A Comprehensive Guide for General Practitioners.* Health professionals worldwide face the challenge daily to manage diabetic patient. This involves not only the treatment of both simple and complex wounds but also engaging with the patient and their families to help prevent injury leading to wounds.

Our knowledge on all aspects of diabetes and diabetic wound management advances every year and it is very important for clinicians to keep up to date with changes in techniques, products, and practice for diabetic patients.

Professor Aziz Nather has, with this new book, provided a very comprehensive text of 20 chapters covering a broad range of topics, chapters, and a supplement of 10 sections with topics including team approach, types of dressings, negative pressure wound therapy, maggot debridement therapy, offloading diabetic foot, hyperbaric oxygen therapy, Charcot joint disease, and rehabilitating diabetic foot.

Professor Aziz Nather has written and edited the publication with contribution from global leaders in the field and doctors from his department. This book is a comprehensive guide for general practitioners who are often presented with patients with diabetic foot problems.

This book will be a valuable addition to the range of publications on diabetes, wound identification and management, and patient education.

This book will be very relevant for general practitioners, nurses, podiatrists, and other health professionals.

Associate Professor Geoff Sussman,
OAM JP FPS FACP FAIPM FAWMA FRVAHJ
Immediate Past President Asia Pacific Association for
Diabetic Limb Problems

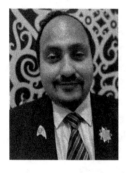

Dear friends and family of the diabetic foot group, it gives me great honour and privilege to write the foreword in yet another amazing book written by none other than Associate Professor Dr. Aziz Nather whom I have known for 20 years. He has been a great source of knowledge and expertise in the Asia Pacific region and has left a big legacy for all of us to follow. He has authored and edited many books.

This book is titled *Understanding Diabetic Foot: A Comprehensive Guide for General Practitioners*. I have the great pleasure of writing one chapter in this book. David Sacketts wrote about Evidence-Based Medicine and Its Importance. Then, we moved on to Evidence-based Practice and Real World Evidence. Clinicians manage diabetic foot patients in a comprehensive and holistic manner. Professor Mike Edmonds propagated the theory of a multidisciplinary team approach for the past 40 years. All this can be summed up into one fact whereby all knowledge has to be imparted to various clinicians, and in this book, the general practitioner is the focus, but this masterpiece can be utilised by a broad range of healthcare professionals.

The gist of this book paints the picture of how to recognise signs and symptoms and when to refer to obtain the best management or standard of care for the patients who are our clients. The most important aspect is to prevent avoidable amputation. Save lives and save limbs is a crucial end outcome in our fight against the diabetic foot syndrome.

In addition, we need books such as this which are filled with loads of experience and information at the fingertips of the primary care doctors in the community as they are the first frontliners in the fight against amputation and limb preservation in diabetes and its complication. I wish Dr. Aziz the very best and record my utmost gratitude to him for continuing to be a teacher and a beacon of hope for the medical fraternity during our hours of need.

Education #Education#Education

Thank you.
Take care and God bless.

Professor Dr. Harikrishna K. R. Nair
President Elect World Union of Wound Healing Societies
Chair, Commonwealth Wound Care Resource Alliance
President Asia Pacific Association for Diabetic Limb Problems
Chairman, ASEAN Wound Council

Preface

This book is the fourth written by the author on "Diabetic Foot", the earlier books being *Diabetic Foot Problems* (2008), *The Diabetic Foot* (2012), and *Surgery for Diabetic Foot* (2016), all books published by World Scientific Publishing Company Private Limited.

It is written as a comprehensive and practical guide for General Practitioners (GPs) who often manage patients with diabetic foot complications. Topics written include types of diabetic foot complications, the basic science involved including the pathogenesis of diabetic foot and the anatomy and biomechanics of the foot, assessment of the diabetic foot, and the holistic treatment of diabetic foot — endocrine control, nutritional control, and choosing the appropriate wound dressing and appropriate antibiotic.

An important chapter, especially useful to GPs is a practical guide on when to treat the patients in their clinics and when to send them to hospitals for management by diabetic foot specialists. A special emphasis has also been given to guide GPs on how to educate their patients on care of diabetes itself, care of the foot, and choice of footwear.

This book will also be useful to other professionals including nurses and podiatrists who also provide care to diabetic foot patients. For the latter professionals, a supplementary section has been added. Relevant topics include team approach, wound dressings, negative pressure wound therapy, maggot debridement therapy, offloading, hyperbaric oxygen therapy, Charcot joint disease, and rehabilitation.

This book will be useful not only to GPs but also to all doctors, medical students, nurses, podiatrists, and other allied health professionals in countries in the ASEAN and Asia Pacific region including Singapore, Malaysia, Indonesia, Thailand, the Philippines, Thailand, Vietnam, Myanmar, India, Pakistan, Hong Kong, China, Taiwan, Japan, and Korea and also in other regions including Europe, the Middle East, Central Asia, and Latin America.

This book will be released in February 2023. It will be officially launched in October 2024 during the 20th Conference of Asia Pacific Association for Diabetic Limb Conference (APADLP) to be held in Singapore in conjunction with the 20th Anniversary of the association. It was set up in Singapore in 2004 with Dr. Nather as the Founding President.

Dr. Aziz Nather
Associate Professor, Author & Editor,
Senior Consultant Orthopaedic Surgeon,
Diabetic Foot Surgeon,
Visiting Consultant, Jurong Medical Centre
National University Health Services, Singapore
Founding President APADLP
Current Honorary Secretary APADLP
Board Member ASEAN Wound Council

About the Editor

Dr. Aziz Nather
Associate Professor & Senior Consultant
Orthopaedic Surgeon
Diabetic Foot Surgeon
Jurong Medical Centre
National University Health Services
Singapore

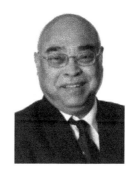

- Chairman, NUH Diabetic Foot Team, May 2003–December 2019.
- Founding President, Asia Pacific Association of Diabetic Limb Problems (APADLP): 2004–2006.
- Current Honorary Secretary, APADLP.
- Board Member, ASEAN wound Council.
- Chairman of the Following Conferences in Singapore:
  - First National & Regional Conference on Diabetic Foot Conference, 2004.
  - 5th Asia Pacific Conference on Diabetic Limb Conference, 2008.
  - 10th Asia Pacific Conference on Diabetic Limb Conference, 2013.
  - 20th Asia Pacific Conference on Diabetic Limb Conference, 2024.
  - 20th Anniversary of APADLP.

- Authored and Edited the Following Books:
  - o Diabetic Foot Problems, World Scientific, 2008
  - o The Diabetic Foot, World Scientific, 2012
  - o Surgery for Diabetic Foot, World Scientific, 2016
  - o Understanding Diabetic Foot: A Comprehensive Guide
  For General Practitioners, World Scientific, 2023

List of Contributors

Editor And Author

Associate Professor Aziz Nather
MBBS (Singapore), FRCS Edin, FRCS Glas, MD (NUS)
Senior Consultant Orthopaedic Surgeon
Diabetic Foot Surgeon
Jurong Medical Centre
National University Health Services
Singapore
Email: Aziznather1973@ gmail.com

Chairman, NUH Diabetic Foot Team
May 2003 to December 2019

Founding President, Asia Pacific Association for Diabetic Limb Problems
(APADLP)
2004 to 2006

Current Honorary Secretary, APADLP

Council Member ASEAN WOUND COUNCIL

Other Authors

Professor Dr. Harikrishna K. R. Nair, MD, FRCPI, FRCP Edin, PG in Wound Healing & Tissue Repair (Cardiff, UK), Ph.D. (Austria), S.I.S KMN

Head & Consultant
Wound Care Unit
Department of Internal Medicine
Hospital, Kuala Lumpur
Professor, Faculty of Medicine
Lincoln University, Malaysia
Email: Hulk25@hotmail.com

President, Malaysian Society of Wound Care Professionals (MSWCP)

President-Elect, World Union Wound Healing Societies (WUWHS)

President, Asia Pacific Association for Diabetic Limb Problems (APADLP)

Chairman ASEAN Wound Council

Chair, Commonwealth Wound Care Resources Alliance

Vice President of D-Foot International

Member, International Surgical Wound Complications Advisory Panel (ISWCAP)

Member, International Wound Infection Institute (IIWII)

National Advisor for Wound Care in Primary Health

Editor-in-Chief, *Wounds Asia Journal*

Editor-in-Chief, *Malaysian Journal of Medical Research*

Gulnaz Tariq, RN, RM, Post Grad (Pakistan), MSc (UK), IIWCC (Toronto)
Stars Medical Assistant Centre
Abu Dhabi
Email: gulnaz.t5@gmail.com

President, World Union of Wound Healing Societies (WUWHS)

CEO International Interprofessional Wound Care Group (IIWCG)

Member, International Surgical Wound Complications Advisory Panel (ISWCAP)

Clinical Advisor Debra Pakistan

Associate Professor Gulapar Srisawasdi, MD, C Ped

Director, Sirindhorn School of Prosthetics and Orthotics
Faculty of Medicine
Siriraj Hospital
Mahidol University
Bangkok, Thailand
Email: gulapar@yahoo.com

President-Elect, Asia Pacific Association For Diabetic Limb Problems

Regional Chairman, Western Pacific Region, D-Foot International

Vice President D-Foot (2018–2020)

Associate Professor Geoffrey Sussman, OAM JP

Associate Professor of Wound Care
Faculty of Medicine, Nursing and Health Science
Monash University
Clinical Lecturer Medical Education
University of Melbourne
Australia
Email: Geoff.sussman@monash.edu

Immediate Past President, Asia Pacific Association For Diabetic Limb Problems

Executive Board Member of International Wound Infection Institute

Executive Board Member of Australasian Wound and Tissue Repair Society

Chairman Wounds Australia Credentialling Committee

Associate Editor of *International Wound Journal*

Dr. Amaris Lim Shu Min, MBBS (Singapore)

Family Medicine Resident Year 3
National University Hospital
1E Kent Ridge Road
Singapore 119228
Email: Amaris_sm_lim@nuhs.edu.sg

Dr. Claire Chan Shu-Yi, MBBS (Singapore)

Resident Year 3
Imperial College London
United Kingdom

10th NUH Diabetic Foot Clinical Research Team 2014

Eda Lim Qiao Yan, MBBS (Singapore)

Wee Lin, MBBS (Singapore)

Zest Ang Yi Yen, MBBS (Singapore)

Joy Wong Ler Yi, MBBS (Singapore)

Department of Orthopaedic Surgery
NUH Diabetic Foot Team
National University Hospital

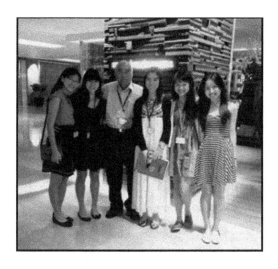

Attached as Clinical Research Assistants
to Associate Professor Aziz Nather in
NUH Diabetic Foot Team —
January to May 2014

11th NUH Diabetic Foot Clinical Research Team 2015

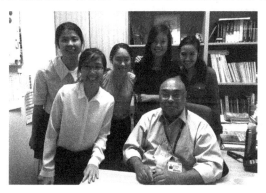

Tan Ting Fang, MBBS (Singapore)

NurAmalina Anwar, MBBS (Sydney)

Julia Cheong Ling-Yu, MBBS (UK)

Department of Orthopaedic Surgery
NUH Diabetic Foot Team
National University Hospital

Attached as Clinical Research Assistants
to Associate Professor Aziz Nather in
NUH Diabetic Foot Team —
January to May 2015

12th NUH Diabetic Foot Team Clinical Research Team 2016

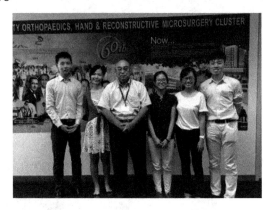

Mae Chua Chui Wei, MBBS (Singapore)

Cao Shuo, BDS (Singapore)

Jere Low, MBBS (Singapore)

Department of Orthopaedic Surgery
NUH Diabetic Foot Team
National University Hospital

Attached as Clinical Research Assistants
to Associate Professor Aziz Nather in
NUH Diabetic Foot Team —
January to May 2016

Lee Jia Hui, Michelle
Staff Nurse
Outpatient Clinic
Department of Orthopaedic Surgery
National University Hospital

Tan Chin Fen
Staff Nurse
Outpatient Clinic
Department of Orthopaedic Surgery
National University Hospital

Contents

Section 1

Introduction to Diabetes

Chapter 1

Diabetes in the World

Aziz Nather and Julia Cheong Ling-Yu

Introduction

Diabetes is one of the fastest growing health challenges of the 21st Century. There is currently 463 million adults living with diabetes. A further 1.1 million children and adolescents live with Type 1 diabetes. 1.6 million deaths are directly attributable to diabetes each year.

IDF[1] estimates that there will be 578 million adults with diabetes by 2030, and 700 million by 2045.

Diabetes Hot Spots in the World

China has the world's most serious diabetes problem, and the problem is escalating drastically. **India** comes next. Together, China and India accounts for more than 40 per cent of the world's population of diabetes today.

Other hot spots include the **Middle East and Central America**.

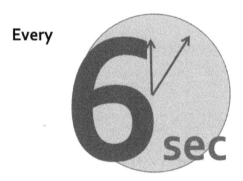

A person dies from diabetes

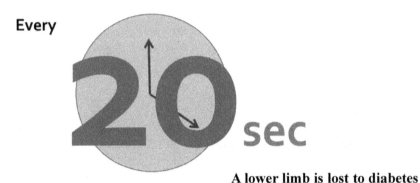

A lower limb is lost to diabetes

In **2019**[2] the estimated global direct health expenditure on Diabetes is **USD 760 billion**.

By **2045**, this is expected to grow to a projected **USD 845 billion** worldwide, an 11.2 % increase.

Global health expenditure due to diabetes

India

Currently, there are about **77 million** diabetics (8.9 %).

By **2045**, the number of diabetics will rise to over **134 million, the second highest number of diabetics worldwide.**

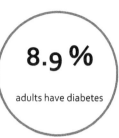

China

116 million individuals suffered from diabetes in 2019 (11.2 %), the **highest** number of diabetics in **the entire world**.

By **2045**, the number of diabetics will increase to **147 million**.

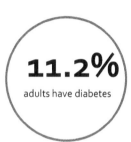

South East Asia

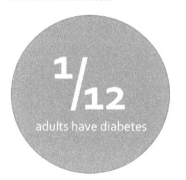

88 million people have diabetes in 2019.

By **2045** the number of people with diabetes is projected to rise to **153 million**.

1 in 2 diabetes patients are undiagnosed *and are at a higher risk of developing harmful and costly complications.*

Singapore

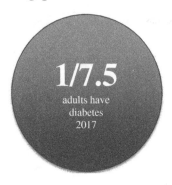

Has one of the **highest prevalence** of diabetes in the developed world **(10.53 % in 2019)**.

In **2019, 640,000** suffered from diabetes, costing **USD 1.34 billion annually**.

If nothing is done, it will increase to **796,000** in **2030** costing an estimated **USD 1.4 billion a year**. It will further increase to **826 million** in **2045**, with an estimated cost of **USD 2.5 billion annually**.

References

1.   IDF Diabetes Atlas*: Ninth edition, International Diabetes Federation* (2019).
2.   *https://www.diabetesresearchclinicalpractice.com*
3.   *The Straits Times. 14 April* 2016.

Chapter 2

Diabetes in Singapore Today

Aziz Nather and Tan Ting Fang

Introduction

Currently, we have more than 640 million adults with diabetes.[1] Singapore has the second largest prevalence of diabetes (10.53 %) among the developed nations, next to the United States (10.75 %).[2] It is costing US$1.34 billion in health expenditure annually, and if nothing is done, it will increase to 796,000 in 2030 costing an estimated US$1.4 billion. It is further projected to be 826,000 in 2045 with an estimated cost of US$2.5 billion annually.

Changing Dynamics

Asians have become more at risk of getting diabetes compared to the other races. This is because as Asians become richer, they "brought in unhealthy Western lifestyle" leading to higher risks of obesity and diabetes.[3]

Facts and Figures (Figure 1 — *Straits Times*, 14 April 2016)

- 1 in 9 Singaporeans is a diabetic.
- 1 in 3 diabetics does not know he or she has diabetes.
- 1 in 2 heart attack patients has diabetes.

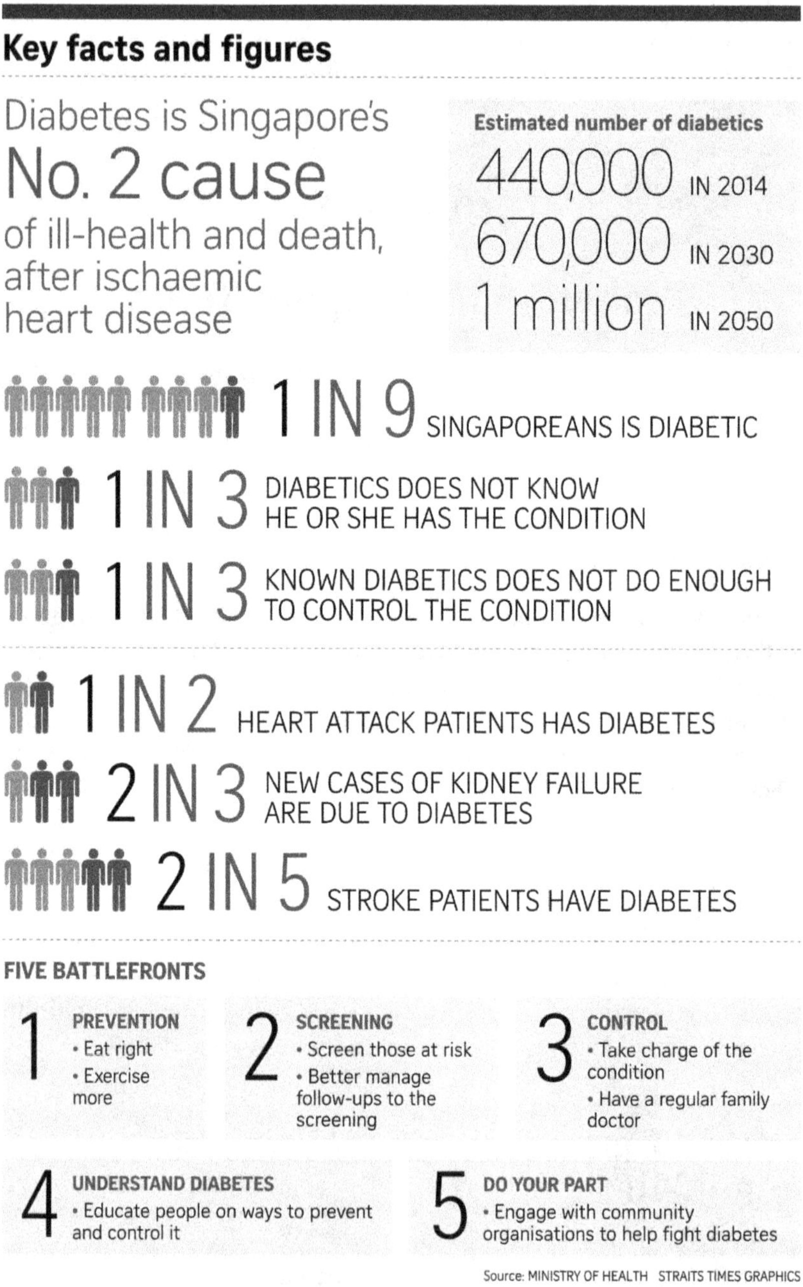

Key facts and figures

Diabetes is Singapore's
No. 2 cause
of ill-health and death,
after ischaemic
heart disease

Estimated number of diabetics

440,000 IN 2014

670,000 IN 2030

1 million IN 2050

1 IN 9 SINGAPOREANS IS DIABETIC

1 IN 3 DIABETICS DOES NOT KNOW HE OR SHE HAS THE CONDITION

1 IN 3 KNOWN DIABETICS DOES NOT DO ENOUGH TO CONTROL THE CONDITION

1 IN 2 HEART ATTACK PATIENTS HAS DIABETES

2 IN 3 NEW CASES OF KIDNEY FAILURE ARE DUE TO DIABETES

2 IN 5 STROKE PATIENTS HAVE DIABETES

FIVE BATTLEFRONTS

1 PREVENTION
• Eat right
• Exercise more

2 SCREENING
• Screen those at risk
• Better manage follow-ups to the screening

3 CONTROL
• Take charge of the condition
• Have a regular family doctor

4 UNDERSTAND DIABETES
• Educate people on ways to prevent and control it

5 DO YOUR PART
• Engage with community organisations to help fight diabetes

Source: MINISTRY OF HEALTH   STRAITS TIMES GRAPHICS

Figure 1:   Key Facts and Figures on Diabetes[2] in Singapore

- 2 in 3 new cases of kidney failure are due to diabetes.
- 2 in 5 stroke patients have diabetes.

From a Ministry of Health viewpoint, it is a good strategy to deal with diabetes early and on a national scale in order to save healthcare expenditure costs.

Parliamentary Debate on Diabetes, 13 April 2016

It is therefore not surprising that on 13 April 2016, in a parliamentary debate, the then Minister of Health (Mr. Gan Kim Yong) "declared War on Diabetes". He set up a new task force to deal with diabetes on "five battlefronts"[2]:

- *Prevention*
  - Eat right
  - Exercise more
- *Screening*
  - Screen those at risk
  - Better manage follow-ups to the screening
- *Control*
  - Take charge of the condition
  - Have a regular family doctor
- *Understand Diabetes*
  - Educate people on ways to prevent and control it
- *Do Your Part*
  - Engage with community organisations to help fight diabetes

War on Diabetes, April 2016

- … The war on Diabetes will not be a quick battle, but a long war requiring sustained effort.
- … Success will be far reaching as it will "curb not just diabetes but other related diseases such as heart disease, renal failure …"
- … "it will improve their lives and reduce the burden on their families."

— **Health Minister, Mr. Gan Kim Yong**

National Day Rally Speech, 2017

The Prime Minister highlighted this serious problem[4]:

> ...."It is because many people are not worried that I am worried. It is precisely because many people do not take diabetes seriously that it has become a very serious problem in Singapore."

> — **PM Lee Hsien Loong, National Day Rally, 2017**

References

1. IDF Diabetes Atlas, *International Diabetes Federation*, 9th Edition (2019).
2. War on Diabetes, *The Straits Times*, 14 April 2016.
3. M.E. Png, J. Yoong, T.P. Phan *et al.*, Current and future economic burden of diabetes among working-age adults in Asia: Conservative estimates for Singapore from 2010–2050, *BMC Public Health* **16**: Article 153 (2016).
4. *National Day Rally*, Prime Minister Office (2017).

Chapter 3

Prevention of Diabetic Foot: Role of Government Intervention

Aziz Nather and Cao Shuo

Diabetic Foot Strategy

Our diabetic foot strategy is two-pronged:

(1) The first strategy is to prevent the development of diabetic foot complications. This is achieved by providing education (90% of prevention) and by performing annual foot screening (10% of prevention).
(2) The second strategy, to be used when prevention fails and a complication develops, is to treat the complication by an Inter-Disciplinary Diabetic Foot Team. We started such a team at the National University Hospital in 2004 coupled with the implementation of a clinical pathway, coordinated by a Clinical Co-ordinator.[1]

Prevention is Key

Prevention is the key to managing diabetic foot problems.10–15% of diabetics develop at least one foot ulcer during their lifetime.[2] 84% of non-traumatic limb amputations in diabetes are preceded by foot ulcers.[3]

The first pillar of prevention is education (90% of prevention). Education needs to be given to patients and caregivers (80% of our efforts) and also to healthcare professionals (20% of our efforts).

The second pillar of prevention is annual foot screening (10% of prevention). This should be provided to all patients newly diagnosed with diabetes. Annual foot screening should be performed in all diabetics along with annual eye, heart, and kidney screening. Lavery *et al.*[4] showed annual foot screening to produce a 47.5% decrease in amputation rate.

Patient Education

Curriculum for Patient Education

Patients must be educated on three topics[5]:

(1) *Care of Diabetes*
    Many patients with diabetic foot do not know or do not care much about diabetes at all. Our first step is to make them understand diabetes and why it is important for them to take care of diabetes.
(2) *Care of the Foot*
    Many patients have poor foot hygiene. Many do not take care of the foot at all.
(3) *Using Proper Shoes for Protection*
    Many patients do not wear protective shoes outdoors. They prefer to walk bare feet. They must learn the importance of protective footwear and how to choose appropriate shoes.

These three topics are discussed in Chapters 17–19.

Education pamphlets on these three topics are found in Appendix of the ASEAN Guidelines for Management of Diabetic Foot Problems, published in the *Sri Lankan Journal Diabetes Endocrinology Metabolism* in 2015.[5] The guidelines were produced by an expert group forum comprising two experts from each country. Participating countries include Indonesia, Malaysia, the Philippines, Singapore, Sri Lanka, and Thailand. The forum is chaired by Dr. Aziz Nather, who also edited the proceedings of the forum. The guidelines were completed and printed in July 2014 for distribution to all six participating countries.

These education pamphlets were designed and printed by National University Hospital (see Chapter 20) in English (Figure 1) and Malay (Figure 2) for giving to our patients in the outpatient clinics and wards.

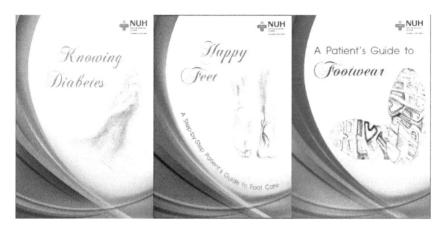

Figure 1:   Education Pamphlets in English

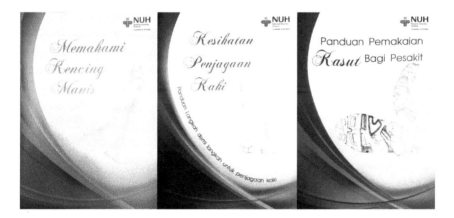

Figure 2:   Education Pamphlets in Malay

Annual Foot Screening

This is described in detail in Chapter 16 on "When to Refer Diabetic Foot Complications."

Role of Government Involvement

Conducting National Public Awareness Programme

The best way to achieve prevention is by conducting a Public Awareness Programme. To be effective, this must be done on a national scale. It is a massive responsibility to target our entire population of 5.7 million. To succeed, we need the government to commit its involvement by forming a Joint Task Force to include the following ministries:

- Ministry of Health
- Ministry of Education
- Ministry of Culture, Community and Youth
- Ministry of Communication and Information
- Ministry of Family Development

Such a task force must also include doctors, nurses, and other allied health professionals at various levels:

- *Primary Health Care Level*: Our doctors and nurses in our nationwide polyclinics.
- *Secondary Health Care Level*: Our doctors and nurses in all major hospitals.

Only a combined Joint Task Force involving all the relevant ministries and health professionals at all levels would be effective in providing public awareness to the whole nation.

National Programme for Public Awareness

This national programme should include the following:

- ***Educational talks to institutions***
  - o   in schools, both primary and secondary,
  - o   in polytechnics and universities.

- Face-to-face talks coupled with free foot screenings
- Currently, with the COVID era, *online talks and webinars*
  - *involve patients* to discuss
    - what they already know,
    - what they don't know and need to know,
    - what they want to know,
    - patient empowerment.
- ***Educational talks on radio and television***
- ***Articles in daily newspapers***
  - *Straits Times, Lianhe Zaobao, Lianhe Wanbao, Shin Min Daily,*
  - *Berita Harian, Berita Minggu, Tamil Murasu, Business Times,*
  - *The New Paper, Today, Weekender, Tabla.*
- ***Advertisements in cinemas and shopping malls***
- ***Advertisements on MRTs, buses, and taxis***

Algorithm for Prevention of Diabetic Foot

Our algorithm for prevention of diabetic foot in Singapore[6] is depicted in
Figure 3. This shows our two main pillars of prevention to be education

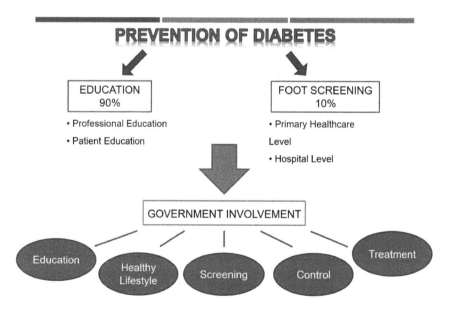

Figure 3:   Algorithm for Prevention of Diabetes in Singapore[6]

(90%) and screening (10%), but central to our success is government involvement. Singapore is fortunate to have our government committed to involvement in the prevention of diabetes in Singapore.

Summary

- The key to management of diabetic foot is prevention.
- The first pillar of prevention is education (90%).
  - o   of patients and caregivers (80% of our education efforts),
  - o   of healthcare professionals (20% of our education efforts),
- The other pillar of prevention is foot screening (10%).
- Central to these two pillars is the third and most important pillar: government involvement.
- This central pillar is essential if success is to be achieved on a national scale.

References

1. A. Nather *et al.*, Value of team approach combined with clinical pathway for diabetic foot problems. A clinical evaluation, *Diabetes Foot Ankle.* **1**: 5731 (2010).
2. G.E. Reiber and W.E. Ledous, Epidemiology of diabetic foot ulcers and amputations: evidence for prevention, in: R. Williams *et al.* (eds.), *The Evidence Base for Diabetes Care,* John Wiley & Sons, London, pp. 641–665 (2002).
3. H. Brem *et al.* Evidence-based protocol for diabetic foot ulcers, *Plast Reconstr Surg.* **117**(7 Suppl): 193S–209S (2006).
4. Lavery *et al.*, Disease management for the diabetic foot: effectiveness of a diabetic foot prevention program to reduce amputations and hospitalisations, *Diabetes Res Clinic Practice.***70**(1): 31–37 (2005).
5. A. Nather *et al.*, Asean plus guidelines for the management of diabetic foot wounds, *Sri Lankan J Diabetes Endocrinol Metab.* **5**(1): 2015.
6. A. Nather *et al.*, Prevention of diabetes, *Singapore Med J* **59**(6): 291–294 (2018).

Chapter 4

Understanding Diabetes

Aziz Nather and NurAmalina Anwar

Diabetes Mellitus is a **chronic** disease. The pancreas does not produce enough insulin (Type 1), or the body does not respond to the insulin it produces (Type 2).

This leads to an increased concentration of glucose in the blood (**hyperglycaemia**).

How Insulin Works?

Normal Individuals

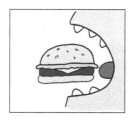 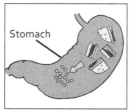 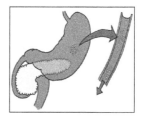

1. After a meal,

2. The food we eat gets digested into glucose.

3. Blood glucose level increases to above normal.

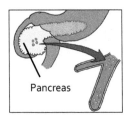 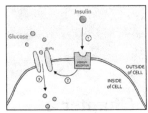 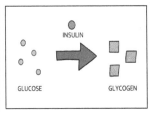

4. The pancreas then secretes a hormone called insulin

5. Insulin enables glucose to enter various cells. Blood glucose level returns to normal.

6. Insulin converts extra glucose into glycogen for storage. Blood glucose level returns to normal.

Did you know?

The normal blood glucose level ranges from *3.5–8.0 mmol/L*

Diabetic Individuals

Type 1

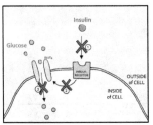

Pancreas produces little or no insulin (insulin deficiency). Blood glucose level remains high, as glucose cannot enter cells or be converted into glycogen.
It usually occurs in children and young adults.

Type 2

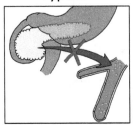

Cells do not respond normally to insulin (insulin resistant). Blood glucose level remains high.
It is usually caused by genetic and environmental factors (e.g. diet & exercise).

Risk Factors

- Obesity (Body Mass Index >25.0)
- High blood pressure
- Family history of diabetes
- Gestational diabetes
- Coronary Heart Disease
- Abnormal fat and cholesterol levels

Symptoms

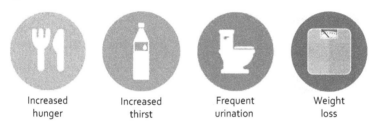

| Increased hunger | Increased thirst | Frequent urination | Weight loss |

Glossary

Medical Term	Definition
Diabetes Mellitus	*A metabolic disease, in which the patient has high blood glucose. Due to inadequate insulin production, or when cells do not respond to insulin.* *It is diagnosed when a patient has* • *Random plasma glucose* > 11.1mmol/L* • *Fasting plasma glucose* >7.0mmol/L* • *Oral glucose tolerance test* >11.1mmol/L*
Random plasma glucose*	*Blood test at any time of the day to measure blood glucose level.*
Fasting plasma glucose*	*Blood test taken after 8 hours of fasting.*
Oral glucose tolerance test*	*Blood test to diagnose diabetes, taken at 1, 2 and 3 hour intervals after drinking glucose.*
Chronic	*Long lasting condition.*
Pancreas	*An organ in the abdomen that produces insulin to regulate the blood glucose level.*

(Continued)

(*Continued*)

Medical Term	Definition
Hyperglycaemia	*An excess of glucose in the bloodstream.*
Glucose	*A type of sugar produced by digestion of food.* *Normal blood glucose concentration:* **3.5–8.0 mmol/L**
Insulin	*A hormone produced by the pancreas that lowers blood glucose level by* • *Promoting entry of glucose into tissue* • *Converting glucose into glycogen*
Body Mass Index (BMI)	$$BMI = \frac{Weight\ (kg)}{Height\ (m)^2}$$ *It is an attempt to quantify the amount of tissue mass (muscle, fat and bone) in a individual, and then categorise that person as* *Underweight (< 18.5)* *Normal Weight (18.5–25)* *Over weight (25–30)* *Obese (>30)*
Gestational diabetes	*When women exhibit high blood glucose levels during pregnancy. No previous diabetes.*
Coronary Heart Disease	*Plaque build-up in the arteries that supplies oxygenated blood to the heart.*
Abnormal fat and cholesterol levels	• *High Density Lipid cholesterol* **<1.0 mmol/l** • *Triglyceride level* **>2.30 mmol/l**

Chapter 5

Complications of Diabetes

Aziz Nather and Tan Ting Fang

Diabetes is a life-long condition that requires careful control. If not, many complications may arise.

Acute Complications

Acute complications are **severe**.

Acidic Blood — Diabetic Ketoacidosis (DKA)

DKA is life-threatening.

It usually occurs in Type 1 diabetes. The accumulation of ketones (products of fat and protein breakdown) acidifies blood. This is toxic to the body.

Symptoms

- Frequent urination
- Always thirsty
- Weight loss
- Nausea and vomiting
- Abdominal pain

- Fatigue and weakness
- Breathlessness
- **Confusion**
- **Disorientation**
- **Exhaustion**

"Thick" Blood — Hyperglycemic Hyperosmolar State (HHS)

HHS is also life-threatening.

It usually occurs in Type 2 diabetes. Excessive loss of fluid causes dehydration and blood becomes concentrated.

Symptoms

- Frequent urination
- Always thirsty
- Weight loss
- Weakness
- Visual disturbances

- Leg cramps
- **Drowsiness, seizures and weakness on one side of the body**
- **Coma**

Low Blood Glucose — Hypoglycaemia

When blood glucose concentration is low: **<3.0 mmol/L**.

It occurs when one

- skips, delays, or consumes insufficient meals,
- increases physical activity,
- is given too much insulin.

Symptoms

- Hunger
- Shakiness
- Anxiety
- Sweating
- Dizziness
- Sleepiness
- Mental confusion
- Weakness

- Headache
- Irritability
- Increased heart rate
- Cold skin
- Double vision
- **Seizures**
- **Coma**
- **Death**

Chronic Complications

Chronic complications occur in patients with a **long duration** of diabetes.

What is atherosclerosis?

It is the **blockage of blood vessels**.

High blood glucose causes deposition of fatty materials (plaques) in blood vessels. This narrows and hardens them, reducing blood flow.

It blocks blood flow to

- Heart
- Brain
- Legs
- Kidneys
- Eyes

Normal artery   *Blocked artery*

Heart Attack — Coronary Artery Disease

Coronary arteries are blood vessels that supply the heart with oxygen and nutrients:

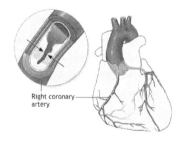

Right coronary artery

- **Partial blockage** of these arteries produces **chest pain**.
- **Complete blockage** results in a **heart attack**.

Symptoms

- Chest pain or discomfort
- Shortness of breath

- Sweating
- Nausea
- Light-headedness

Stroke

This occurs when blood supply to the brain is compromised.

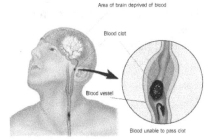

The two most common types are as follows:

- **Stroke**
  One part of the brain dies from lack of blood and oxygen.
- **Mini-stroke** — *Transient Ischaemic Attack (TIA)*
  Temporary fall in blood and oxygen supply can cause brief symptoms of stroke.

Symptoms

- Sudden weakness or numbness on one side of the body
- Sudden confusion
- Sudden difficulty in talking or understanding
- Sudden dizziness, loss of balance, or trouble walking
- Sudden visual disturbances, such as double vision
- Sudden severe headache

Leg Pain — Peripheral Arterial Disease (PAD)

Lack of blood and oxygen to leg muscles, causing pain when walking (vascular claudication) or even at rest (rest pain).

PAD increases the risk of amputation.

Symptoms

- Weak or tired legs
- Difficulty walking or balancing
- Cold and numb feet or toes
- Slow-healing sores and ulcers
- Foot pain at rest
- Leg pain after walking a fixed distance
- Black skin on feet or toes (gangrene)
- Loss of hair, shiny skin, nail changes, and darkened skin

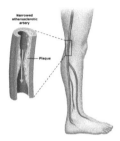

Kidney Damage — Diabetic Nephropathy

Reduced blood flow and damage to the kidney make it less able to filter waste and in severe cases, fail.

There are usually no symptoms until almost all function of the kidney is gone.

Symptoms

- Swelling around the eyes, abdomen, legs, ankles, and feet
- Urination problems e.g. unable to pass urine or passing urine more frequently
- Sallow appearance of face
- Fatigue
- Insomnia
- Breathlessness
- Loss of appetite
- Metallic taste in the mouth
- Nausea or vomiting
- Weakness
- Dizziness
- High blood pressure
- Itching or rashes

Eye Problems — Diabetic Retinopathy

High blood glucose damages small blood vessels in the **retina**. This causes blurred vision or even blindness.

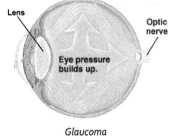

Glaucoma

It may also lead to the following:

- **Cataract**
  Clouding of the lens of the eye can cause blurred vision.
- **Glaucoma**
  Buildup of pressure in the eye can damage the **optic nerve** and lead to blindness.

Symptoms

- Blurry or double vision
- Rings, flashing lights, or blank spots
- Dark or floating spots
- Pain or pressure in one or both eyes
- Difficulty seeing things out of the corners of the eyes

Nerve Damage — Diabetic Neuropathy

Excess blood glucose can injure the walls of tiny blood vessels that supply the nerves, resulting in nerve **ischemia** and damage.

Symptoms

- Numbness, tingling, or pain in the toes, feet, hands, and fingers
- Weakening of muscles in feet or hands

Diabetic Foot Complications

Diabetic patients are more prone to infections due to poor immunity. In addition, wounds take a longer time to heal due to poor blood supply. The foot complications are described in Chapter 6.

Glossary

Medical Term	Definition
Acute	Severe but temporary
Ketoacidosis	Condition when ketone bodies accumulate and acidify the blood
Atherosclerosis	Deposition of fatty materials in blood vessels that narrows and hardens blood vessels, causing blockage
Rest pain	Pain experienced when in rest position (sitting or lying)
Retina	Lining at the back of the eye, detecting light entering the eye
Iris	Coloured portion of the eye
Optic nerve	Nerve carrying images from the eye to the brain

Ischemia	Decreased blood supply to a tissue resulting in shortage of oxygen and glucose to the cell
Inflammation	Part of the body's immune response
Pus	Collection of white blood cells, dead cells, and bacteria

Section 2

Introduction to Diabetic Foot

Chapter 6

Types of Diabetic Foot Complications

Aziz Nather

Introduction

When diabetes is not controlled properly, a foot complication can develop, just like stroke, heart attack, or renal impairment.

Pathophysiology

Three risk factors may operate to cause a diabetic foot wound. These factors are neuropathy, vasculopathy, and immunopathy — **the "Diabetic Foot Triad"** (Figure 1). Each factor may operate in varying degrees in different patients.

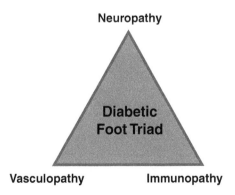

Figure 1:   Diabetic Foot Triad

Neuropathy

Refers to the numbness in the foot that occurs when excess blood glucose damages the nerves in the foot.

Vasculopathy

Refers to blockage of the arteries in the leg — anterior tibial artery or posterior tibial artery that supplies blood to the dorsum (front) or volar aspect (sole) of the foot leading to ischaemia in the foot.

Immunopathy

Refers to the increased susceptibility of the foot to infection when blood glucose is not well controlled.

In some cases, only one risk factor predominates e.g. in dry gangrene due to vasculopathy alone. In others, a combination of two risk factors may be responsible e.g. in wet gangrene due to vasculopathy with superimposed infection (immunopathy). In still other cases, all three factors may contribute: neuropathy, vasculopathy, and immunopathy.

Before a doctor can treat the problem successfully, he must first carefully examine the patient's foot to assess the risk factors present. Treatment must involve addressing the risk factors that operate.

Types of Diabetic Foot Problems

Skin Infection — Cellulitis

It is the **inflammation** of the skin.

The skin is red, painful, warm, and tender (Figure 2).

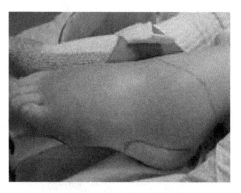

Figure 2 :   Cellulitis

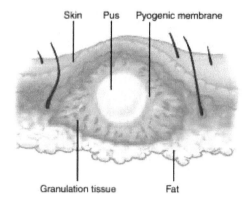

Figure 3:   Abscess

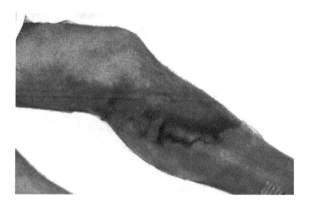

Figure 4:   Necrotising Fasciitis

Abscess

It is an accumulation of **pus** beneath the skin (Figure 3). The foot is swollen, red, and painful.

Necrotising Fasciitis

It is the most dangerous diabetic foot infection (Figure 4) — also known as a "flesh-eating" disease.

It is caused by infection spreading rapidly beneath the skin on the covering of muscle.

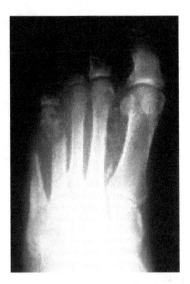

Figure 5:   Osteomyelitis of Fourth Metatarsal Head

The patient looks ill and febrile, and has severe pain and tenderness in the foot.

X-rays show gas under the skin. It has a high mortality rate of 20–40%.

Bone Infection — Osteomyelitis

It is an infection of the bone and bone marrow (Figure 5). It is identified by deep tenderness of the infected bone when touched.

It is important to diagnose it early to avoid limb amputation.

Joint Infection — Septic Arthritis

This is an infection of adjacent bones and the joint involved. It occurs commonly in the metatarsophalangeal joints (MTPJs) of the foot (Figure 6).

Movement of the affected joint causes severe pain. The range of motion of the joint is also severely restricted.

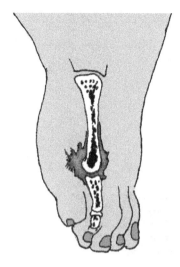

Figure 6:   Septic Arthritis of 4th MTPJ

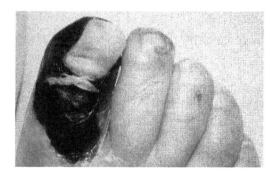

Figure 7:   Wet Gangrene Big Toe

Dead Tissue — Gangrene

It occurs due to the lack of blood supply to the toes and feet. It presents as blackening of the toes or heel:

- **dry** gangrene — uninfected dead tissue,
- **wet** gangrene — infected dead tissue (Figure 7). Note cellulitis adjacent to big toe gangrene.

Joint Breakdown — Charcot Joint Disease

It is a progressive condition that causes deformity in the foot (Figure 8).

Progression:

1. Joint Breakdown
2. Bone Destruction (Figure 9)
3. Deformity

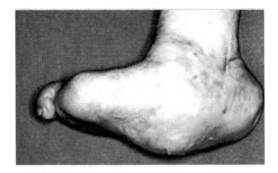

Figure 8:   Rocker Bottom Foot

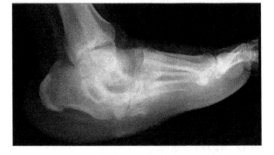

Figure 9:   Bone Destruction in Midfoot

Ulcers — Wounds

Breakdown of skin showing the underlying tissue.
    Ulcers can be

• infective,
• ischaemic,

- neuropathic (no sensation),
- decubitus (due to pressure).

Infective Wound

This is due to infection. Signs of infection are present. The floor of the ulcer usually shows slough and some pus or exudate. The adjacent skin of the wound shows signs of inflammation with adjacent cellulitis.

It usually occurs on the dorsum of the foot (Figure 10), in the web space or on the heel.

It can also occur in the sole of the foot.

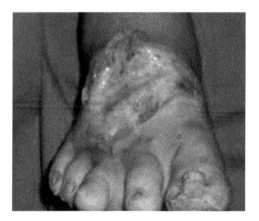

Figure 10:   Infective Ulcer Over Dorsum of Foot with Slough and Pus with Adjacent Cellulitis

Ischaemic Wound

This is due to ischaemia (Figure 11). The involved foot may show signs of chronic ischemia: shininess of the skin, increased skin pigmentation, trophic nail changes, and loss of hair.

There is reduced perfusion in the foot. One or both foot pulses may not be palpable. Capillary refill in the toes is poor (less than 2 seconds). The foot is cold and pale looking. The edge of the wound is necrotic.

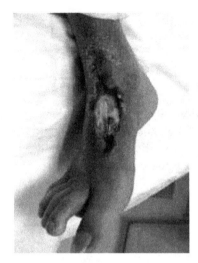

Figure 11:   Ischaemic Ulcer on the Dorsum of Foot with Necrotic Edge. Dorsum Foot is Dusky in Colour

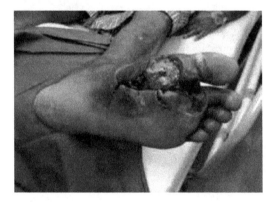

Figure 12:   Infective and Ischaemic Wound in the Sole of Foot

Both Infective and Ischaemic

Some wounds have features of both infection and ischaemia (Figure 12).

Neuropathic Wounds

These usually occur in weight-bearing areas of the foot (Figures 13 and 14) as a result of loss of protective sensation (neuropathy) and high pressure

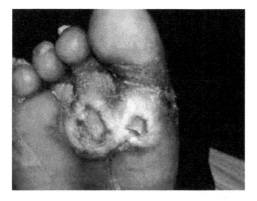

Figure 13:   Neuropathic Ulcers in Sole Over First and Second Metatarsal Heads

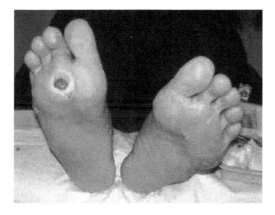

Figure 14:   Neuropathic Ulcer in Sole Over Second Metatarsal Head

points in the foot due to altered biomechanics. Examination reveals the presence of sensory neuropathy with a reduced feeling to pinprick, loss of vibration sense, and position sense.

Pressure Wounds

These occur in a bedridden or wheelchair-bound patient when excessive pressure is placed on the skin over a prolonged duration of time. The common sites include the areas over the lateral malleolus (Figure 15) and the lateral aspect of the base of the fifth metatarsal and the back of the heel (Figure 16).

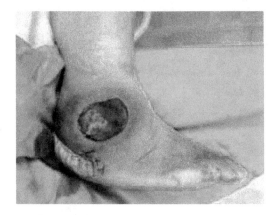

Figure 15:   Pressure Ulceration Over Lateral Malleolus

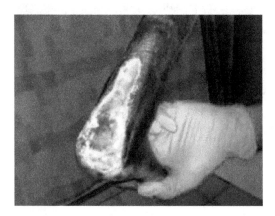

Figure 16:   Pressure Ulceration Over Back of Heel

Classifying the Diabetic Foot Wound

It is useful to classify wounds because this reflects the severity of and extent of the wound in question. This is useful for communication with the doctor in the hospital.

A simple classification system to use is the Wagner–Meggitt classification system[1,2] (Table 1 and Figure 17). This classification is easy to use and is popularly used by medical students.

Table 1:   Wagner–Meggitt Classification System

Grade	Description of ulcer
Grade 0	Pre- or post-ulcerative lesion completely epithelialised
Grade 1	Partial/full-thickness ulcer confined to the dermis, not extending to the subcutis
Grade 2	Ulcer of the skin extending through the subcutis with exposed tendon or bone; no abscess formation or osteomyelitis
Grade 3	Deep ulcer with abscess formation or osteomyelitis
Grade 4	Localised gangrene of the toes or partial foot gangrene
Grade 5	Whole foot gangrene

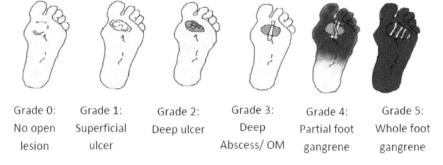

| Grade 0: | Grade 1: | Grade 2: | Grade 3: | Grade 4: | Grade 5: |
| No open lesion | Superficial ulcer | Deep ulcer | Deep Abscess/ OM | Partial foot gangrene | Whole foot gangrene |

Figure 17:   Wagner–Meggitt Classification System

References

1. B. Meggitt, Surgical management of the diabetic foot, *Br J Hosp Med.* **16**: 227–232 (1976).
2. F.W. Wagner, The dysvascular foot: a system for diagnosis and treatment, *Foot Ankle.* **2**(2): 64–122 (1981).

Chapter 7

Know Your Foot: A Simple Guide to Anatomy and Biomechanics of the Foot

Aziz Nather and Julia Cheong Ling-Yu

Introduction

The feet are flexible structures comprising bones, joints, muscles, and ligaments that help us stand, walk, run, and jump.

The Anatomy

Bones of the Leg

- Bones of the leg support the many muscles that allow us to carry out all sorts of activities (e.g. walking and running).
- They must be strong enough to support our body weight while remaining flexible enough for movement and balance.

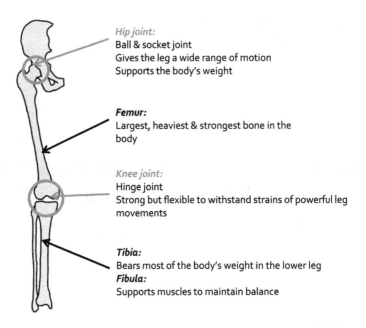

Hip joint:
Ball & socket joint
Gives the leg a wide range of motion
Supports the body's weight

Femur:
Largest, heaviest & strongest bone in the body

Knee joint:
Hinge joint
Strong but flexible to withstand strains of powerful leg movements

Tibia:
Bears most of the body's weight in the lower leg
Fibula:
Supports muscles to maintain balance

Bones of the Foot

There are three sections in a foot:

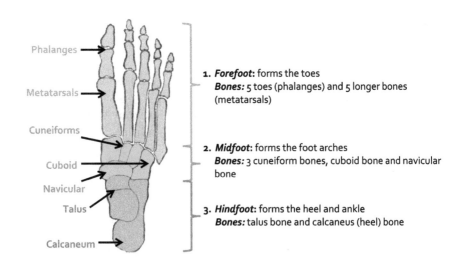

Phalanges

Metatarsals

Cuneiforms

Cuboid

Navicular

Talus

Calcaneum

1. **Forefoot:** forms the toes
   Bones: 5 toes (phalanges) and 5 longer bones (metatarsals)

2. **Midfoot:** forms the foot arches
   Bones: 3 cuneiform bones, cuboid bone and navicular bone

3. **Hindfoot:** forms the heel and ankle
   Bones: talus bone and calcaneus (heel) bone

Did you know?

- There are **26 bones** and **33 joints** in the foot
- The **largest** bone in the foot is the **calcaneus (heel) bone**

Muscles of the Lower Leg

- Our leg muscles are responsible for supporting, balancing, and propelling our body.
- There are three main groups of muscles in the lower leg:

Lateral: Works together to plantar flex foot (e.g. standing on your toes) and bend (flex) toes.

Posterior: Works together to plantar flex foot.

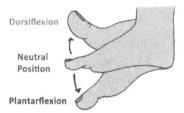

Dorsiflexion

Neutral Position

Plantarflexion

Anterior: Works together to dorsiflex foot and straighten (extend) toes.

Muscles of the Foot

- Help support arches of the foot and control toe movement.

Did you know?

There are **more than 100** tendons, ligaments and muscles in the foot

Dorsal extensor muscles:
Extensor muscles are located on the top (dorsal side) of the foot

- Control straightening of toes

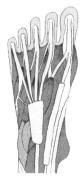

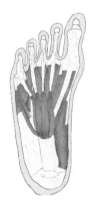

Plantar flexor muscles:
Flexor muscles are located on the sole (bottom or plantar side) of the foot

- Control bending of toes

Blood Vessels of the Leg and Foot

- Blood vessels carry vital oxygen and nutrients to nourish tissues in the leg (arteries) and remove carbon dioxide and waste produced by tissues in the leg (veins).
- There are three main arteries that supply blood to the foot.

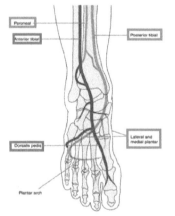

Posterior tibial artery and peroneal artery:
- Form **lateral and medial plantar arteries** in foot.
- Supply blood to **bottom** of foot and toes.

Anterior tibial artery:
- Forms **dorsalis pedis** in foot.
- Supplies blood to **top** of foot.

The main vein in the leg and foot is the **great saphenous vein**.

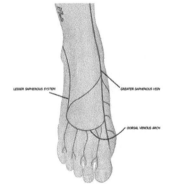

Nerves of the Foot

There are two main nerves in the foot:

○ ***Medial plantar nerve***
○ ***Lateral plantar nerve***

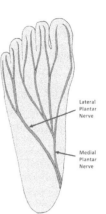

- Send and receive signals for locomotion (movement) and balance of the body.
- Control muscles of the feet to create constant, slight shifts to prevent us from falling down.

How We Walk — The Gait Cycle

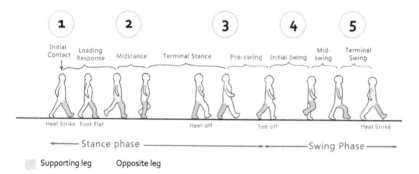

1 Stance phase
Contact phase: Heel strike (contact with ground) → foot flat (entire foot on ground)

2 Mid-stance phase: Foot flat → mid-stance (opposite foot heel-off) → toe-off (opposite foot)

3 Propulsion phase: Heel-off (supporting foot) → toe-off (supporting foot) + heel strike (opposite foot)

Swing Phase

4 Acceleration → mid-swing: Toe-off (supporting foot) → moving limb gains speed

5 Mid-Swing → Deceleration: Moving limb slows down → heel strike (supporting foot)

The cycle repeats.

Glossary

Extensor	Muscles that extend and straighten joints
Flexor	Muscles that bend joints
Gait cycle	Describes how humans walk. It consists of two phases: the stance phase and the swing phase
Stance phase	Phase during which the foot is touching the ground
Swing phase	Phase during which the foot does not touch the ground

Section 3

Assessing Diabetic Foot

Chapter 8

Examining Diabetic Foot in Your Clinic

Aziz Nather

Introduction

In examining a Diabetic Foot Problem (DFP), one must

- take a comprehensive medical history,
- perform a systematic meticulous examination.

History Taking

It is important to take a detailed and complete medical history.

Patient Profile

What is the Patient's Profile?

Patients are usually in the fifth and sixth decades of life.[1] Males and females are equally affected.[1]

What is the Patient's Socioeconomic Status?

There is a higher incidence of DFPs in Malays and Indians as compared to the ethnic–racial composition in Singapore. The incidence in Chinese was significantly lower.[2] They mainly occur in the lower socioeconomic group. Patient's education level is usually up to secondary school only. They tend to have a low average monthly household income of less than SG$2000.[2]

Symptoms

Where is the Pain?

Localise the site of the pain:

- Toe(s)
- Dorsum of foot
- Sole of foot
- Heel

Is There Vascular Claudication?

Vascular claudication is pain in the calf muscle after the patient walks a characteristic claudication distance due to inadequate blood flow. The pain disappears in a few minutes when he stops walking. Vascular claudication, a common symptom of ischaemic limb, is not common in DFPs.

Is There Rest Pain?

Rest pain is common in patients with DFPs. It refers to continuous pain in the distal part of the limb: toes or forefoot. This continuous, severe, and aching pain often stops him from walking and sleeping. It is a symptom of severe or critical ischaemia. The patient usually hangs the leg over the side of the bed. Putting the leg below the level of the heart allows the blood to gravitate into the limb and offers some relief from pain. He prefers to sleep in a sitting position rather than lying on the bed. Sometimes, the rest pain is so severe that the patient begs for an amputation.

Is There swelling?

In cellulitis, the generalised swelling in the foot is associated with redness, warmth, and pain (Figure 1). A localised swelling is usually due to an abscess or infection of the underlying bone (osteomyelitis).

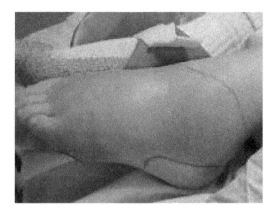

Figure 1: Cellulitis

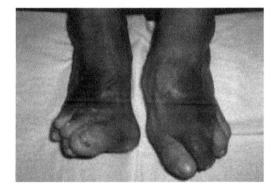

Figure 2: Bilateral Deformed Feet

Swelling of a joint with pain on motion of the joint is usually due to septic arthritis. This commonly involves the metatarsophalangeal joints (MTPJs) of the foot.

Fever, chills, and rigours may be present. Elderly patients and patients with diabetes are usually immunocompromised. Usually, no systemic response is seen in these patients.

Is There Deformity?

Clawing of toes may be present due to motor neuropathy. A large swollen foot with deformity is due to Charcot Joint Disease (CJD). CJD can also be bilateral (Figure 2). Deformity can lead to a loss of the arch of the foot. This can progress to develop a rocker bottom foot deformity (Figure 3).

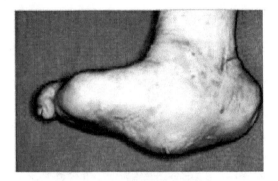

Figure 3:   Rocker Bottom Deformity

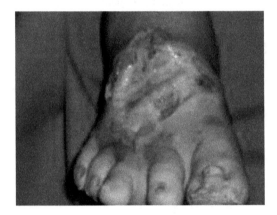

Figure 4:   Ulcer of Dorsum of Foot Showing Infection and Slough

Is There an Ulcer?

An ulcer is one of the commonest presenting symptom in diabetic foot.

Site of Ulcer

Localise the site of the ulcer:

- Dorsum of foot (Figure 4)
- Sole of foot (Figure 5)
- Lateral malleolus
- Heel

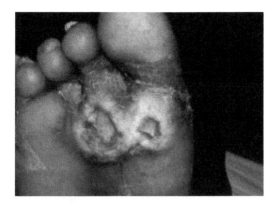

Figure 5:   Ulcer on Sole of Foot (Neuropathic Ulcer)

Contents of Ulcer

Note also the colour and smell of the discharge.

Staphylococcus *aureus*	Thick, brown, little odour
Pseudomonas *aeruginosa*	Greenish, rotten fruit smell, or "metallic" smell
Bacteroides *fragilis* (anaerobe)	"Faecal" smell

Is There Gangrene?

Gangrene is the death of tissue due to lack of blood flow or a serious bacterial infection.

Identify the type of gangrene:

Dry gangrene (Figure 6)	No superimposed infection
Wet gangrene (Figure 7)	With superimposed infection

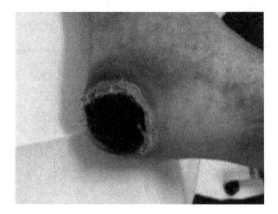

Figure 6:   Dry Gangrene of Heel

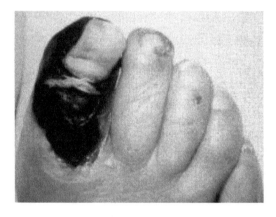

Figure 7:   Wet Gangrene of Big Toe

Ask the patient whether it is painful or not. Usually, pain is felt at the junction of dead and living tissues.

Is There Numbness?

Look for sensory disturbance. It usually presents as "gloves and stocking" distribution on both feet.

How Severe is the Numbness?

If numbness is present, evaluate its severity. Nather used a simple grading system to assess the severity of the numbness based on the type and extent of numbness present (see Nather's Grading System for Numbness described later in the section on Assessment for Neuropathy). The longer the duration of diabetes, the higher the incidence of neuropathy and the higher the grade likely to be present.

Has the Patient had Recent Trauma?

Trauma is usually sustained at home (e.g. when the patient kicks the side of the bed or slips and falls in the bathroom). Often, trauma goes unrecognised because the patient has sensory neuropathy.

Has the Patient Sustained Self-inflicted Trauma?

Cutting of a callosity or digging of a toenail using non-sterile equipment at home.

Does the Patient Self-medicate?

Many patients like to self-medicate. Malays tend to apply coffee powder on their ulcers, Indians apply turmeric, and the Chinese apply herbs from traditional Chinese medicine to heal their wounds. Such applications can cause infections.

What is the Type of Footwear Worn?

Note the type of footwear worn by the patient. Stone *et al.*[3] found that about 70% of diabetics do not wear shoes outside the house. They only wear slippers.

It is important to note the type of slippers worn:

- Japanese slippers put the first web space in jeopardy — ulceration of the first web space.
- Slippers with dorsal straps and ankle straps — ulceration of the dorsum of the foot or the back of the ankle.

Medical History

What is the Type of Diabetes Mellitus Present?

Most patients have Type 2 diabetes (non-insulin-dependent diabetes).

What is the Type of Diabetic Medication Used?

Record diabetic medications employed:

✓ Diabetic diet
✓ Oral hypoglycaemic agents
✓ Oral drugs supplemented with insulin injections

Does the Patient Monitor His Diabetes?

Record the type and frequency of monitoring by the patient:

✓ Urine dipstick
✓ Capillary blood glucose level monitoring

Does the Patient Know His HbA1C Level?

HbA1C level reflects control of diabetes over the last 3 months: HbA1C<7% is good.

What are the Symptoms of Poorly Controlled Diabetes?

The symptoms are polyuria (passing urine frequently and at night), polydipsia (always feeling thirsty), and polyphagia (always feeling hungry).

What are the Complications of Diabetes Present?

Complications	Symptoms
Cataracts	Impairment of vision
Diabetic retinopathy	Damage to retina

Diabetic nephropathy	Sallow appearance
Diabetic neuropathy	"Glove and stocking" sensory disturbance in feet
Diabetic vasculopathy	Vascular claudication or rest pain

What are the Co-morbidities Present?

- Hypertension
- Ischaemic heart disease
- Chronic renal failure
- Cerebrovascular accident (CVA)

Diabetes + Hypertension: Diabetes and hypertension each predispose to atherosclerosis (blockage of arteries). This combination causes an increased risk of peripheral vascular disease with a greater risk of below-knee amputation.

Diabetes + Renal Failure: Diabetes and renal failure each cause immunocompromise. This combination gives a poor prognosis, as the patient is "double-immunocompromised". Healing is delayed.

Diabetes + CVA: This combination also gives a poor prognosis. Severely disabled patients are more prone to pressure ulcerations and to bedsores.

Are Risk Factors of Diabetes Present?

- Hypertension
- Smoking
- Hyperlipidaemia

Social History

What is the Functional Status of the Patient?

- Walker
  - housebound walker
  - community walker

- o   with aid: stick/frame
- o   needs assistance
- Wheelchair-bound
- Bedridden

What is the Patient's Occupation?

- High-Risk Jobs
  - o   Taxi driver, bus driver, lorry driver
  - o   Housewife, cook
  - o   Manual labourer, factory worker wearing safety boots

Is There a Family History of Diabetes?

One parent/both parents/sibling(s)/aunty/uncle.

What is the Lifespan of Family Member with Diabetes?

If the family member died at the age of 88, the chance of the patient living to 70 years or beyond is good.

Is There a Caregiver?

Spouse/daughter/daughter-in-law/sister/aunty/domestic helper.
    The presence of a caregiver is important to provide support to the patient including helping to change dressings.

Performing the Clinical Examination

- Wear
  - o   short-sleeved shirt (or roll-up long-sleeved shirt),
  - o   bow tie (or remove long tie),
  - o   remove watch/bracelet.
- Wash hands with Hibiscrub or perform hand rub with alcohol before and after examining the patient.
- Wear gloves to remove the dressing and to examine the ulcer present.

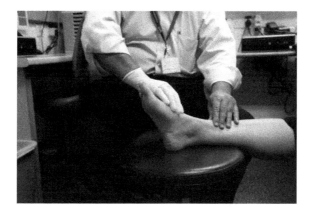

Figure 8:   Position of Patient in the Clinic

Position of Patient

• Put the patient's foot on a stool (Figure 8).
  Examine the foot in seated position.

Perform Step-by-Step Examination

Perform the examination in a systematic manner — step-by-step:

• General examination
• Local examination
  o   assess vascular status
  o   assess sensory neuropathy
  o   assess immunopathy

General Examination

• Is the patient toxic, anxious, or well?
• Is he febrile? Record temperature.
• Is he alert or drowsy due to hypoglycaemia or ketoacidosis?
• Is there acidotic breathing due to ketoacidosis?
• Is there a sallow appearance due to renal impairment?
• Is there pallor? Depress the eyelid and inspect the conjunctiva).

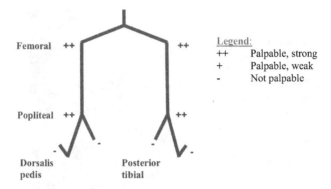

Figure 9:   Pulses in Lower Limb

- Is there dehydration? Ask the patient to stick out his tongue and look for dryness.
- Examine the eyes for cataracts. Is the patient able to read newspapers?
- Examine the sclera for jaundice.

Vital Signs

- Measure blood pressure on both arms
  o   Look for postural hypotension (sudden fall in blood pressure).
- Record pulse rate
  o   Look for tachycardia.
- Record respiratory rate
  o   Look for tachypnoea.
- Palpate all pulses
  o   carotid, axillary, brachial, radial, ulnar, abdominal aorta, femoral, popliteal, dorsalis pedis, and posterior tibial.

Record findings in the stick diagram shown in Figure 9.

Examine Cardiovascular System

- Locate apex beat.
- Look for cardiomegaly.
- Listen for murmurs.

Examine Respiratory system

Look for

- bronchopneumonia,
- pulmonary effusion,
- chronic obstructive lung disease.

Examine Abdomen

Look for

- peritonitis,
- hepatosplenomegaly,
- enlarged bladder.

Local Examination

Before starting, wear gloves. Remove the dressing and place the exposed limb on a clean towel (Figure 10). Place soiled dressing in a plastic bag for disposal.

Inspection

Perform local inspection in a systematic fashion step by step:

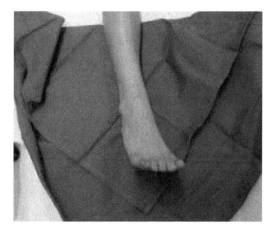

Figure 10: Foot Placed on Sterile Dressing Towel for Examination

- toes/toenails/web spaces,
- dorsum foot,
- sole of foot,
- heel.

Start with examining the toes first. End with examining the heel. Look for

- callosity,
- blister,
- ingrown toenail,
- cellulitis,
- abscess,
- ulcer,
- wet gangrene,
- dry gangrene,
- charcot joint disease.

Palpation

- It is important to palpate the foot.
- Is the redness in the foot warm (infection) or cold (ischaemia)?
- Is there underlying induration or fluctuancy (abscess)?
- Is there crepitus (indicating gas)?

Examining an Ulcer

Examine the wound (Figure 11) using the following protocol:

- **Site**
- **Size**
- **Edge**: incised, everted, inverted, ischaemic
- **Floor**: slough, granulation tissue, tendon, capsule
- **Content**: exudate, pus
- **Environment**: cellulitis of adjacent skin

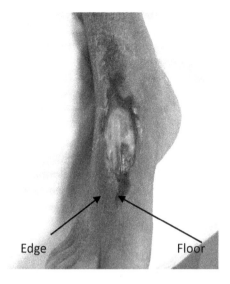

Figure 11:   Ischaemic Ulcer

Assessing Diabetic Foot Triad

One then proceeds to assess the three components of the diabetic foot triad:

- Vasculopathy
- Neuropathy
- Immunopathy

Assessing Vasculopathy

- **Colour of Skin**
  - o   Pink: Normal
  - o   Pale: Ischaemia
- **Temperature of Skin**
  - o   Warm: Normal
  - o   Cold: Ischaemia
- **Pulp Capillary Refill**
  - o   <2 Seconds: Normal
  - o   >2 Seconds: Delayed (Ischaemia)
- **Pulses**

Femoral Pulse

- Midway between pubic tubercle and anterior superior iliac spine (the mid-inguinal point).
- Easiest pulse to feel.

Popliteal Pulse

- Flex the knee to 90 degrees. Place both thumbs on either side of the tibial tuberosity and the other fingers on the popliteal fossa. Relax the hamstrings. Gently press the popliteal artery against the tibia to feel the pulse.
- More difficult to feel (deep-seated).

Dorsalis Pedis Artery (Figure 12)

- Mid-point of anterior ankle line between the medial malleolus and the lateral malleolus (Point A). Drop a line between this point to the first interdigital cleft (Figure 13). The dorsalis pedis pulse can be felt one-third down this line from the anterior ankle line (Point B).

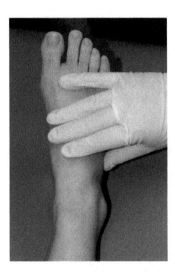

Figure 12:   Palpation of Dorsalis Pedis Artery

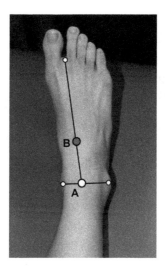

Figure 13: Point A: Midpoint of Line between Malleoli, Point B: 1/3 down the Line from A to First Interdigital Cleft

Posterior Tibial Artery (Figure 14)

- Place the hip in external rotation, the knee in flexion, and the foot in dorsiflexion.

    The landmarks are as follows:

- one-third along the line between the tip of the medial malleolus and the Tendo Achilles (Point C),
- one-third along the line between the tip of the medial malleolus and the point of the heel (Point D) (Figure 15).

Pulses	Type of Surgery That Could Be Performed
2 pulses palpable	• Distal amputation can be performed • Very good chance of success (70–80%)
1 pulse palpable	• Distal amputation can be performed • Fairly good chance of success
No pulse palpable	• Distal amputation should not be performed • No chance of success • Refer to vascular surgeon • Below-knee amputation should be performed if revascularisation fails

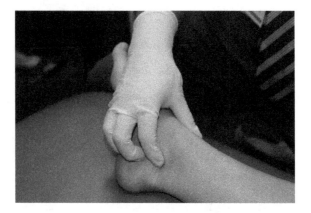

Figure 14:   Palpation for Posterior Tibial Artery

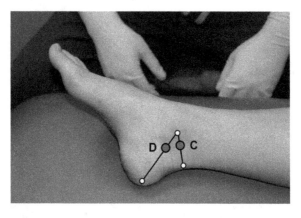

Figure 15:   Showing Points C and D

Assessment for Sensory Neuropathy

1. Pinprick test
2. Position sense test
3. Vibration sense test
4. Monofilament test (optional)

Pinprick Test

Use a pin (neurotip) to test for pain sensation (Figure 16). Sensory disturbance usually occurs in a "glove and stocking" distribution. Assess

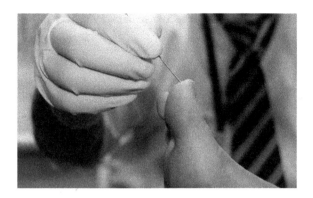

Figure 16:   Pinprick Test

the severity of numbness present according to the type of numbness present.

Map out the extent of the sensory disturbance present. Assess the severity according to the extent of numbness present. Grade the severity of the numbness following a Simple Grading System used by Nather (Table 1).

Position Sense

Hold the sides of the big toe. Move the toe up and down (Figures 17 and 18).

Vibration Sense

Use a 128-Hz tuning fork (Figure 19):

- Place the tuning fork over the bony prominence (tip of toe, medial malleolus, and tibial crest).
- Record whether the patient feels vibration or not.

Ten-Points Semmes Weinstein Monofilament Test (SWMT) (Optional)

Use a 5.07-gauge nylon monofilament to test for touch sensation.

Table 1:   Nather's Grading System for Severity of Numbness

A. Type of Numbness Present	Grading of Numbness
Pins and needles (paraesthesia)	Mild
Increased sensitivity to pain (hyperaesthesia)	Mild
Decreased sensitivity to pain (hypoaesthesia)	Moderate
No pain	Severe
B. Extent of Numbness Present	**Grading of Numbness**
In toes only	Mild
Up to midfoot	Mild
Up to ankle	Moderate
Up to mid-shin or beyond	Severe

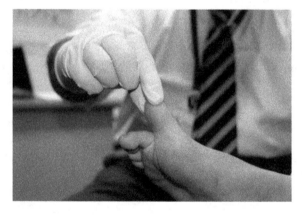

Figure 17:   Position Sense Test, Hallux Dorsiflexion (Up)

Method:

1. Apply monofilament gently over each point and press until it buckles (10-gram force) with the patient's eyes closed (Figure 20).
2. Record "Yes" or "No" for each point.
3. Complete 10 sites of testing (Figure 21).

Normal: $^8/_{10}$ or more sites.

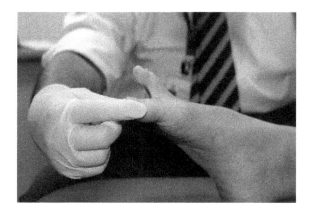

Figure 18: Position Sense Test, Hallux Plantar Flexion (Down)

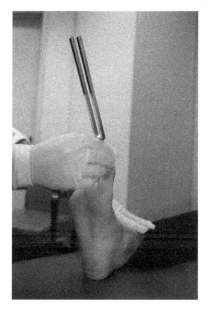

Figure 19: Vibration Sense Test Using 128 Hz Tuning Fork

Abnormal: 7/10 or less sites.

A positive monofilament test is more accurate than pinprick, vibration sense, and position sense combined to detect sensory neuropathy.[4]

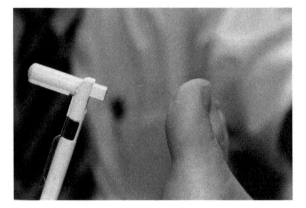

Figure 20:   10 Gram of Force Applied Until filament Bends

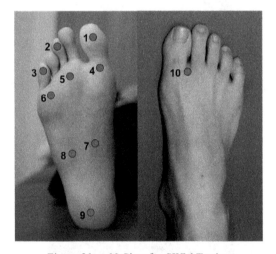

Figure 21:   10 Sites for SWM Testing

Assessment for Immunopathy

Look for

- deep abscess,
- osteomyelitis,
- septic arthritis.

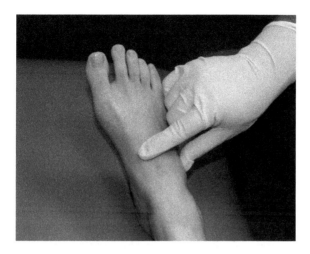

Figure 22:   Deep Palpation Ray by Ray: Dorsum

1. Start on the dorsum of the foot. Move interphalangeal joints and MTPJ gently of the first ray.
2. Look for pain on movement of joints. Severe pain indicates septic arthritis.
3. Perform deep palpation of the bones in the first ray from the distal phalanx, proximal phalanx, and metatarsal to the tibia (Figure 22).
4. Look for tenderness.
5. Next, palpate ray by ray (second, third, fourth, and fifth).
6. Press between first ray and fifth ray.
7. Repeat deep palpation on the sole of the foot (Figure 23).

Most common joints involved in septic arthritis are MTPJs of the foot (Figure 24).

Most common bones involved in osteomyelitis are in the "tripod of the foot": first metatarsal head, fifth metatarsal head, and calcaneum — the weight-bearing points in the Foot.

In necrotising fasciitis (Figure 25), the underlying skin shows cellulitis. In delayed cases, hemorrhagic blisters are classical.

Signs:

*   Look for severe tenderness and tension of the underlying deep fascia.
*   Look for subcutaneous crepitus.

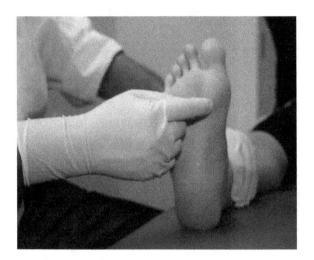

Figure 23: Deep Palpation Ray by Ray: Sole

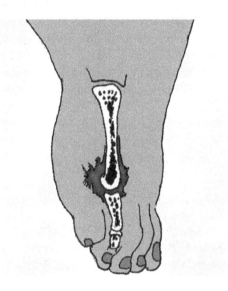

Figure 24: Septic Arthritis of 4th MTPJ

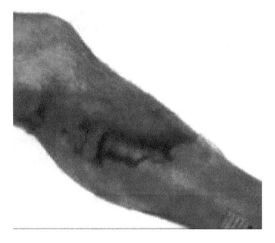

Figure 25:   Necrotising Fasciitis of Leg with Hemorrhagic Blisters

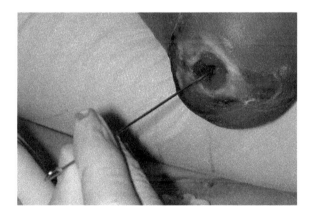

Figure 26:   Probe Test

Probe Test

Put a sterile metal probe into the ulcer (Figure 26). If it reaches the bone, the bone is osteomyelitic.

References

1. A. Nather, S.B. Chionh *et al.*, Epidemiology of diabetic foot problems and predictive factors for limb loss, *J Diabetes Complications.* **22**: 77–82 (2008).
2. A. Nather, S.B. Chionh *et al.*, Socioeconomic profile of diabetic patients with and without foot problems, *Diabetic Foot & Ankle.* **1**: 5523 (2010).
3. K. Stone, A. Nather, Z. Aziz, and A. Erasmus, Footwear in patients with diabetic foot problems, in: *35th Annual General Meeting of Malaysia Orthopaedic Association*, Miri, Sarawak, Malaysia (12 May 2005).
4. G.M. Caputo *et al.*, Assessment and management of foot disease in patients with diabetes, *N Engl J Med.* **331**(13): 854–860 (1994).

Chapter 9

Investigating Diabetic Foot in Your Clinic

Aziz Nather

Introduction

After examining your patient in your clinic, you may need to perform some investigations. These may include blood tests, culture and sensitivity tests, and plain radiographs of the foot.

Blood Tests

In the clinic, when a patient presents with a suspected infection, you may want to perform blood tests.

Markers of Infection

- White Blood Cell (WBC) count
- Erythrocyte Sedimentation Rate (ESR)
- C-Reactive Protein (CRP)

When infection is present, these three markers will be raised. WBC >10,000/L; ESR >20; CRP >20.

At the same time, it is also useful to perform:

Markers of Healing

- HbA1c
- Hb
- Creatinine
- Albumin

When an ulcer is being treated, these markers are useful to predict the chances of healing of the ulcer. Endocrine control must be good for healing to occur — HbA1c must be less than 7%. Enough oxygen must be carried in the blood — Hb must be more than 10 g/dL. Renal impairment impairs healing — creatinine must be less than 90 μmol/L. There must also be enough proteins — albumins must be more than 48 g/L.

Markers of Infection

- ***Full blood count***: A small sample of blood is taken from the vein in the arm.

	Normal Range
WBC	3.40–9.60×10^9/L
Haemoglobin (Hb)	Male: 12.9–17.0 g/dL Female: 11.3–13.5 g/dL

Leukocytosis — when WBC $>10.00 \times 10^9$/L indicates the presence of infection.

- ***Acute phase reactants***:

	Normal Range
ESR	5–15 mm/h
CRP	0–10 mg/L

- *Urea and electrolytes*:

	Normal Range
Urea	2.0–6.5 mmol/L
Sodium (Na)	135–150 mmol/L
Chloride (Cl)	98–107 mmol/L
Potassium (K)	3.5–5.0 mmol/L
Creatinine (Cr)	50–90 μmol/L

- *HbA1c*:

	Normal Range
Patients without diabetes	3.5–5.5%
Patients with diabetes	<7.0%

Total proteins:

	Normal Range
Albumin	38–48 g/L

Culture and Sensitivity (*c/s*) Studies

- *Blood for c/s*
  This procedure is done under sterile conditions. It is done in all cases — even in the absence of a spike in fever. This is because elderly and diabetic patients often have infection without systemic response.
- *Swab for c/s*
  A swab is taken from the ulcer or pus discharged from a wound. Culture is done for both aerobic and anaerobic organisms. The sensitivity of organism(s) present to various antibiotics is performed.

Taking a wound swab
- Take a culture before antibiotics are started.
- Clean the ulcer and the surrounding skin with normal saline.

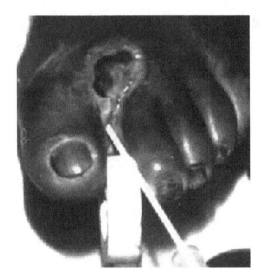

Figure 1:   Wrong Way of Taking A Swab. Swab Stick is Applied to Edge of Ulcer Instead of Centre of Ulcer

- Press the wound at the edges to squeeze the pus out from the centre portion.
- Take the swab from the deepest portion of the ulcer, not from the edges (Figure 1) to avoid contamination by commensals harboured in the neighbouring skin.
- Send the swab for c/s for aerobic and anaerobic organisms.

- *Taking a tissue specimen*
  A tissue specimen is preferred to a wound swab. However, in a clinic setting, this cannot be done.
      Tissue specimen is preferred and done in the treatment room in a hospital outpatient clinic or even better in the operating theatre.

Radiological Tests

- *Radiographs of the foot*: Anteroposterior (AP) and oblique views (Figure 2(a) and 2(b)) for a lesion in the forefoot or midfoot.
- *Radiographs of the ankle*: AP and lateral views (Figure 3(a) and 3(b)) for a lesion in the hindfoot.

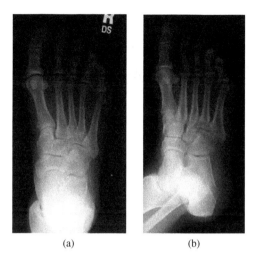

Figure 2: (a) and (b) AP and Oblique Views of Foot

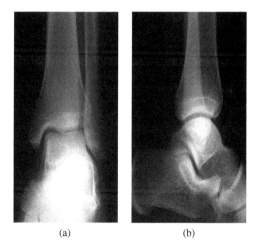

Figure 3: (a) and (b) AP and Lateral Views of Ankle

Look for the following features:
- loss of soft tissue plane,
- calcification of vessels: dorsalis pedis (DP) or posterior tibial (PT) artery (Figure 4(a)),
- erosion of adjacent bone abutting a joint: septic arthritis (Figure 4(b)),

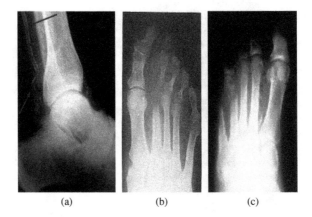

(a)   (b)   (c)

Figure 4:   (a) Calcification of Posterior Tibial Artery. (b) Erosion of Second Metatarsal Head and Adjoining Base of Proximal Phalanx with Septic Arthritis of Second Metatarsophalangeal Joint. (c) Pathological fracture of Fourth Metatarsal Bone Due to Osteomyelitis and Gas Shadows Between Third and Fourth Rays Due to Necrotising Fasciitis

- erosion of bone: osteomyelitis (Figure 4(c)),
- presence of gas: serious life-threatening infection — necrotising fasciitis (Figure 4(c)),
- dislocation of joint, bone destruction: Charcot Joint Disease (CJD).

Chapter 10

Recognising Osteomyelitis in Diabetic Foot

Aziz Nather and Claire Chan Shu-Yi

Introduction

Osteomyelitis (OM): infection of bone and bone marrow is a common complication of diabetic foot. It occurs in 15% of diabetic foot ulcers and in 20% of diabetic foot infections.[1] It is frequently missed and underdiagnosed in patients with diabetic foot problems. A high index of clinical suspicion is required to make a diagnosis. Yet it is very important to suspect and recognise OM early and refer to hospital as soon as possible as undiagnosed it often leads to the dreaded complication of limb amputation. The risk for amputation in acute diabetic infections is four times higher with OM than with soft tissue infection alone.[2]

Location

The most common bones involved are the weight-bearing bones of the foot — the "tripod of the foot"[3] (Figure 1):

- first metatarsal head,
- fifth metatarsal head,
- calcaneum.

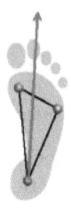

Figure 1:   Weight-bearing Tripod of Foot

In patients who are wheelchair bound, it involves the lateral decubitus bones[3]:

- lateral malleolus,
- base of fifth metatarsal bone,
- calcaneum.

Clinical Examination

There are two scenarios:

- When bone is exposed in a wound, that bone is osteomyelitic unless proven otherwise.
- When the bone underlying the wound is painful and tender, suspect OM.

Deep palpation of the foot ray by ray reveals tenderness of the involved bone (first or fifth metatarsal head or calcaneum). In septic arthritis, movement of the joint is painful (first or fifth metatarsophalangeal joint).[3]

Probe-to-bone Test

In an ulcer, if a clean pip stick reaches the bone, OM is present (Figure 2).[4]

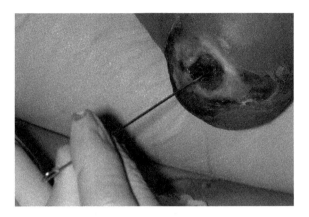

Figure 2:   Probe Test

OM in a Non-healing Ulcer

If an ulcer takes a long time to heal, you must suspect OM to be present. Perform deep palpation for bone tenderness and perform X-rays. You may also decide to refer the patient to a hospital for evaluation and treatment.[3]

Investigations

When you suspect OM, you may perform the following investigations.

Blood Investigations

These include the following:

Markers of infection

- WBC: >15,000
- CRP: >100
- ESR

For more details, refer to Chapter 9.

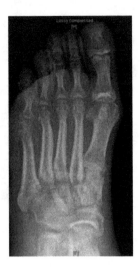

Figure 3:   AP View of Foot Showing Bone Destruction in Fifth Metatarsal Bone Head

Plain Radiographs

- X-rays of foot — AP and oblique views: For ulcer in forefoot or midfoot.
- X-rays of ankle — AP and lateral views: For lesion in hindfoot.

Look for the following changes:

- Periosteal reaction
- Radiolucency
- Area of bone destruction (Figure 3)

Note that radiographic changes may only be visible about 2 weeks after the bone infection occurs.

High Index of Suspicion

A high index of suspicion is required to diagnose OM.[3] It should be suspected when there is the following:

- Severe infection and foot is red, swollen, and tender
- Bone tenderness underlying an ulcer

- Bone is exposed in a wound
- Probe Test is positive and
- Markers of infection are markedly raised
  o WBC >15,000
  o CRP >100
- X-rays show erosive changes in bones
- Or in a chronic ulcer refusing to heal for more than 4 weeks

It is important to diagnose it early and to treat it promptly to obtain a good outcome and give the patient a good prognosis. Delay can lead to the dreadful outcome of a limb amputation.[3]

References

1. S.D. Ramsey *et al.*, Incidence, outcomes, and cost of foot ulcers in patients with diabetes, *Diabetes Care.* **22**: 382–387 (1999).
2. L.A. Lavery *et al.*, Risk factors for developing osteomyelitis in patients with diabetic foot wounds, *Diabetes Res Clin Pract.* **83**: 347–352 (2009).
3. R. Malhotra, C.S.Y. Chan, and A. Nather, Osteomyelitis in the diabetic foot, *Diabetic Foot Ankle.* **5**: 24445 (2014).
4. G.M. Caputo *et al.*, Current concepts: assessment and management of foot disease in patients with diabetes, *New Engl J Med.* **331**: 854–860 (1994).

Section 4

Treating Diabetic Foot

Chapter 11

Treating Diabetic Foot: A Holistic Approach

Aziz Nather

Introduction

In treating a diabetic foot ulcer, one must provide holistic treatment. We must treat the whole patient and not just the foot problem.

Holistic Treatment

This includes the following:

- Ensuring good endocrine control
- Providing nutritional support
- Performing wound bed preparation
  - time concept
  - conventional dressings
  - NPWT and NPWTi
- Administering appropriate antibiotics
- Performing surgery when needed
  - debridement/SSG
  - distal (minor) amputation
    - ray/trans-metatarsal/Pirogoff amputation
  - proximal (major) amputation as a last resort,

- when all attempts to achieve limb salvage fails
- below-knee amputation
- must avoid "creeping amputation"

In this chapter, we will only discuss medical treatment. Surgical treatment will be briefly described in a separate chapter.

Endocrine Control

Poor glycaemic control is common in patients with diabetic foot ulcers.[1]
Factors that contribute include the following:

- Infection
- Stress

One must ensure that good glycaemic control is achieved to allow the ulcer to heal.

Targets:

- Pre-meal Glucose   7.2 mmol/L
- HbA1c   8%

If glycaemic control is poor in a patient on oral hypoglycaemics, optimise by adding Insulin.
The patient should have an HbA1c of less than 8% to ensure good healing of the wound.

Nutrition

Good nutrition is important for wound healing.[1] Proteins are needed in the healing process. It is therefore important that we advise the patient to maintain a healthy and balanced diet. Table 1 summarises the markers of healing.

Table 1:   Markers of Healing

Markers of Healing	Recommended Value	Normal Value
HbA1c	<8%	6.5–8%
Haemoglobin (Hb)	>10 gm/dL	12–16 gm/dL
Total Albumin	>35 gm/L	35–50 gm/L

Anaemia is a common finding in the elderly. Oxygen carried in the blood by haemoglobin will convey the much-needed oxygen to the tissues. If Hb is <10, oxygen carried to the wound is insufficient. If anaemia is present, this needs to be corrected. Likewise, if albumin is less than 5 gm/L, this must also be addressed by giving a high-protein diet.

In addition, vitamin C (ascorbic acid) and zinc are also important elements to facilitate wound healing. Oral vitamin C tablets of 1,000 mg should also be prescribed. This tablet also contains 10 mg zinc citrate trihydrate.

Wound Bed Preparation

Wound bed preparation is important to promote healing of wounds.[2] Important aspects include the following (Figure 1):

- Debridement of wounds
- Managing the bacterial burden
- Managing the exudate

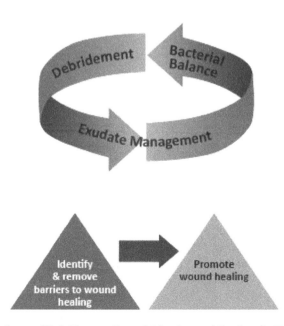

Figure 1:   Balance of Debridement, Bacterial burden, and Exudate for Wound Healing

Time Concept

Use time concept for wound bed preparation[1] (Figure 2, Table 2).

Types of Dressings

The type of dressing to be chosen depends on the level of exudate in the wound and whether there is an infection or not (Table 3, Figure 3).

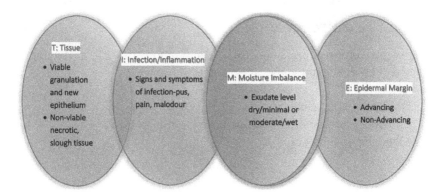

Figure 2:   TIME Concept

Table 2:   Action Needed Following TIME Concept

Clinical Observation	Action Needed
T Tissue non-viable	Debridement
I Infection	Remove infected focus
	Use antimicrobial dressing
M Moisture imbalance	Apply moisture-balancing
• Dessication	Dressing
• Maceration of wound margin	Apply foam dressing
E Edge of wound	
• Non-advancing	NPWT/SSG
• Undermining	Debridement

Table 3:   Simple Guide to Choose Wound Dressing

Characteristic(s) of Wound	Recommended Category Of Dressing
Low exudate	Hydrocolloid, hydrofibre
Dry necrotic wound	Hydrogel
Moderate exudate	Alginate
Moderate to heavy exudate	Foam
Infected wound	Antimicrobial • Silver dressing • Iodine dressing

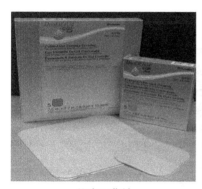

Hydrocolloid

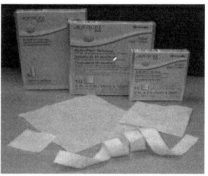

Hydrofibre

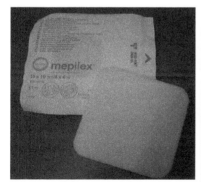

Foam

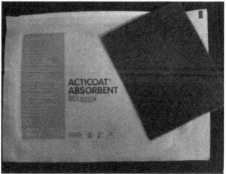

Antimicrobial

Figure 3:   Types of Dressings

Negative Pressure Wound Therapy and Negative Pressure Wound Therapy with Instillation

Negative Pressure Wound Therapy (NPWT)[1] (Figure 4) is useful for the following:

- large wounds e.g. after debridement for necrotising fasciitis,
- wounds which after debridement show exposed tendons, joint capsules, or bone.

NPWT promotes angiogenesis and the formation of granulation tissue. It is useful for wound bed preparation. Once the wound bed is

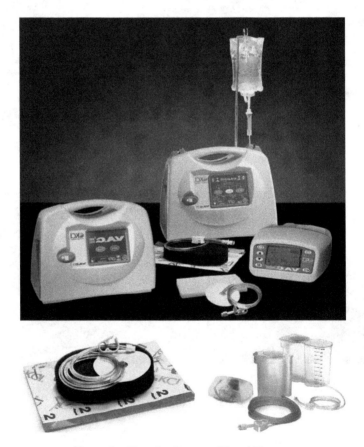

Figure 4:   Negative Pressure Wound Therapy

adequately prepared, it should be stopped and Split Skin Grafting (SSG) performed. This saves time and costs. It usually takes a longer time to wait for the wound to contract completely with just NPWT alone.

Negative Pressure Wound Therapy (NPWTi) with Instillation is a useful adjunct to be used for infective wounds. After debridement and there is still some residual pus, NPWTi could be used for irrigation with just normal saline. The key to NPWTi is the use of special granufoam with large pores allowing for saline to be instilled into the wound and for exudate to perfuse out of the wound. Once the effluent is clear, NPWTi can be stopped and converted to NPWT till it is again ready for SSG.

Antibiotics

It is important to use antibiotics appropriately and judiciously.[1]

The following are useful tips to consider:

(1) Take a swab for C/S BEFORE starting on an antibiotic.
(2) Start with an appropriate first-line antibiotic.

AUGMENTIN is usually taken as the first-line antibiotic — 625 mg bd.

This is because it covers a broad spectrum of organisms — both Gram-positive cocci and Gram-negative rods and some anaerobes. It has the disadvantage of pseudomembranous colitis as a side effect. It is also not effective against pseudomonas.

If a particular organism is strongly suspected to be present, the appropriate antibiotic may be chosen instead and started first until the C/S results return (Table 4).

Table 4:   Choice of First-Line Antibiotic

Characteristics of Discharge	Likely Micro-organism	Recommended Antibiotic
Brownish white, thickish discharge minimal odour	Staphylococcus *aureus*	Cloxacillin 500 mg6H
Greenish discharge, rotten fruit odour	Pseudomonas *aeruginosa*	Ciprofloxacin 500 mg BD
Faecal foul-smelling odour	Anaerobe • Bacteroides • Peptostreptococcus	Flagyl 500 mg (7.5 mg/kg) 6H

(3) Trace C/S results usually back by 3 days and alter the antibiotic(s) if needed based on confirmed bacteria identified.

(4) Avoid using topical antibiotic cream — bactroban cream, polymyxin cream, or neomycin cream to avoid the risk of developing antibiotic resistance.

References

1. ASEAN Plus Guidelines. *Management of Diabetic Foot Wounds*. Section 3 Medical Treatment. July 2014.

2. R.G. Sibbald, D. Williamson, H.L. Orsted, *et al*. Preparing the wound bed-debridement, bacterial balance and moisture balance, *Ostomy Wound Manage* **46**: 14 (2000).

Chapter 12

Antibiotics for Diabetic Foot Infections: A Practical Guide for the General Practitioner

Aziz Nather and Amaris Lim Shu Min

Introduction

Diabetic foot infections are common complications of poorly controlled diabetes. Nather *et al.*[1] showed that infection occurred in 122 out of a cohort of 202 patients with diabetic foot problems (60.4%). Of these, 63 patients (31.2%) had monomicrobial infections and 59 patients (29.2%) had polymicrobial infections.

Diagnosis

Skin and Soft Tissue Infections

All wounds are colonised by micro-organisms but not all of them are infected. A wound infection is defined by the presence of at least two of the following clinical findings:[2]

- local swelling or induration,
- erythema,
- local tenderness or pain,

- local warmth,
- purulent discharge.

In cases of peripheral neuropathy or ischemia, the above local inflammatory signs may be diminished. There should be a high clinical suspicion of infection in wounds that are healing poorly or have necrotic or friable granulation tissue.

Osteomyelitis

Osteomyelitis refers to infection of the bone, with the involvement of the bone marrow. It may occur even without evident soft tissue infection. Osteomyelitis commonly involves the weight-bearing bones of the foot, the "Tripod of the foot", namely the first metatarsal head, fifth metatarsal head, and the calcaneum.

The following clinical signs should raise suspicion for osteomyelitis:

- wounds that are healing poorly,
- exposed bone in the floor of the wound,
- probe-to-bone test positive,
- point tenderness on palpation of the bone.

These patients should be referred to the hospital for further evaluation and treatment.

Local Microbiological Data

In a study completed in 2011, Nather *et al.* analysed a cohort of 100 patients treated for diabetic foot infections.[3] 48% of the infections were monomicrobial while 52% of the infections were polymicrobial.

The most common pathogens found in all infections were as follows:

- Staphylococcus *aureus* (39.7%),
- Bacteroides *fragilis* (30.3%),
- Pseudomonas *aeruginosa* (26.0%),
- Streptococcus *agalactiae* (21.0%).

Mild infections tend to be monomicrobial infections, which are predominantly caused by Gram-positive cocci.

Severe infections are usually polymicrobial. While Gram-positive cocci still predominate in such infections, Gram-negative rods and/or anaerobes are also usually involved.

Collection of Specimen for Culture

As all wounds are colonised with micro-organisms, wound samples should only be sent for culture when there is a clinical suspicion for infection.

Obtaining a specimen for culture prior to starting antibiotics helps identify the causative pathogen, ensuring that antibiotic therapy is targeted and effective. While tissue samples are the preferred specimens for culture, wound swabs can be taken in the primary care setting where wound debridement and tissue sample collection are not possible.

Collecting a Wound Swab

1. Clean the wound with cotton balls or gauze soaked in normal saline.
2. A no-touch technique is preferred if possible — hold the cotton balls with forceps instead of with gloved hands.
3. Extend the tip of the swab into the wound to swab the base of the wound.
4. Avoid touching the edges of the wounds or the skin margins, as the surface of the wound is usually colonised by micro-organisms that may not be a reliable representation of the true pathogens causing deeper infection.
5. Remove the stopper from the tube (Figure 1) and insert the swab into the transport medium. Screw the top on tightly.

In abscess, the aspirate should be sent for culture. In a case of suspected osteomyelitis, upon admission to the hospital, a bone sample obtained in a sterile manner is preferred. Blood cultures should also be done for systemically unwell patients.

Specimen should ideally be taken for culture prior to initiating empirical antibiotics. Administering antibiotics prior to collection of specimen for culture results in lower sensitivity and poorer yield of culture results. However, in systemically unwell patients or in cases where the limb is threatened, the initiation of antibiotics should not be delayed.

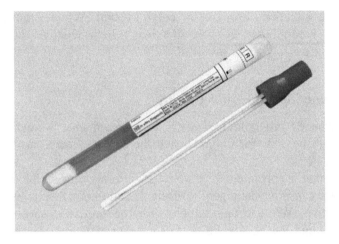

Figure 1:   Culture Medium

Severity of Infection

Accurate assessment of the severity of diabetic foot infections has significant implications on the prognosis and management of the infections.

The IWGDF[4] and IDSA[2] have published guidelines outlining the classification of diabetic foot infections according to levels of severity (Table 1).

Outpatient Management of Diabetic Foot Infections

Mild diabetic foot infections can be managed in the outpatient setting conservatively (Table 2). These patients should be treated with oral antibiotics, regular wound dressings, and off-loading pressure around the wound. Topical antibiotics are not recommended for the treatment of mild diabetic foot infections.

Antibiotics should not be started for wounds that are not infected with the aim of promoting wound healing or for prophylaxis against infection. Overtreating with antibiotics can lead to higher rates of antibiotic resistance in the local population.

Table 1:   IWGDF and IDSA Classification of Diabetic Foot Infections

Clinical Manifestation of Infection	IWGDF Grade	IDSA Infection Severity
No symptoms of signs of local infection: • Local swelling or induration • Erythema • Local tenderness or pain • Local warmth • Purulent discharge	1	Uninfected
At least two of these items are present: • **Local swelling or induration** • **Erythema >0.5 cm around the wound** • **Local tenderness or pain** • **Local increased warmth** • **Purulent discharge** And no other cause of an inflammatory response of the skin (e.g. trauma, gout, acute Charcot neuro-osteoarthropathy, fracture, thrombosis, or venous stasis)	NA	Infected
Local infection with no systemic manifestations (see the following): • **with erythema that does not extend >2 cm around the wound** • **involving only the skin and the subcutaneous tissue (without involvement of deeper tissues and without systemic signs as described in the following)**	2	Mild
Local infection with no systemic manifestations (see the following): • **with erythema >2 cm OR** • **involving structures deeper than skin and subcutaneous tissues (e.g. abscess, osteomyelitis, septic arthritis, and fasciitis)**	3	Moderate
Local infection (as described above) with the signs of SIRS, as manifested by ≥2 of the following: • **Temperature >38°C or <36°C** • **Heart rate >90 beats/min** • **Respiratory rate >20 breaths/min or $PaCO_2$ <32 mmHg** • **White blood cell count >12,000 or <4000 cells/μL or ≥10% immature (band) forms**	4	Severe

Table 2:   Summary Guide for Outpatient Management of Mild Diabetic Foot Infection

Blister	Oral antibiotics
	De-blister if painful
	Regular wound dressings
Ingrown toenail	Oral antibiotics, analgesia
	Place cotton floss under corner of toenail that is cutting into skin
	Footwear with wider toe boxes
	If persistent or worsening, can consider referral to polyclinic or orthopaedic clinic for wedge resection.
Cellulitis	Oral antibiotics
	Offloading of foot
	Elevate limb
	If no improvement, or patient turns systemically unwell, refer to ED for intravenous antibiotics and closer monitoring.
Superficial wounds (fulfilling criteria for IWGDF Grade 2 or IDSA mild infections)	Send wound swab/tissue for culture
	Oral antibiotics
	Offloading of foot
	Regular dressings
	If no improvement, or patient turns systemically unwell, refer to ED for intravenous antibiotics and closer monitoring.
Small abscess <2 cm	Trial of oral antibiotics
	Offloading of foot
	Close monitoring with early review within 3–5 days
	If no improvement, refer to ED for incision and drainage.

Choosing the Antibiotic Regimen

Once a wound culture has been taken, an empirical antibiotic regimen can be implemented based on local microbiological data. A more definite antibiotic regimen can be decided after tracing wound culture results.

Amoxicillin/clavulanate is a good choice of antibiotic for mild diabetic foot infections due to its broad-spectrum coverage against Gram-positive cocci, Gram-negative rods, and even some anaerobes. Cloxacillin and cephalexin are also suitable agents for coverage of Gram-positive cocci. In patients with penicillin allergy, clindamycin or levofloxacin may be considered.

Empirical antibiotics can also be selected based on what the most likely pathogen might be. This can sometimes be deduced from clinical findings, especially the characteristics of the wound discharge (Table 3).

Table 3:   Selection of Empirical Antibiotics Based on Wound Discharge

Characteristics of Discharge	Likely Micro-organism	Recommended Regimen
Brownish discharge Minimal odour	Staphylococcus *aureus*	Cloxacillin 500 mg6H
Greenish discharge Odour of rotting fruits	Pseudomonas *aeruginosa*	Ciprofloxacin 500 mg BD
Faecal foul-smelling odour	Anaerobes	Amoxicillin/clavulanate 625 mg TDS AND Flagyl 500 mg (7.5 mg/kg)6H

Table 4:   Summary of Recommended Empirical Antibiotics for Diabetic Foot Infections

	Mild	Moderate to Severe
Types of wounds	Cellulitis Infected wounds/ulcers with erythema extending <2 cm, involving only the skin and the subcutaneous tissue	Infections with erythema extending >2 cm or involving structures deeper than skin and subcutaneous tissues Patients with signs of SIRS
Microbiology	Gram-positive cocci	Gram-positive cocci Gram-negative rods Anaerobes +/− multi-drug resistant organisms
IDSA Guidelines (2012)[2]	Dicloxacillin Clindamycin Amoxicillin/clavulanate Cephalexin Levofloxacin	Levofloxacin Cefoxitin Ceftriaxone Ampicillin/sulbactam Moxifloxacin Ertapenem Imipenem/cilastatin Tigecycline Levofloxacin/ciprofloxacin + clindamycin
IWGDF Guidelines (2020)[4]	Penicillin 1st generation cephalosporins	Amoxicillin/clavulanate 2nd and 3rd generation cephalosporins

(Continued)

Table 4   (*Continued*)

Mild	Moderate to Severe
Penicillin allergy: Clindamycin, fluoroquinolones, trimethoprim/ sulfamethoxazole, macrolides	Recent antibiotic treatment: Piperacillin/tazobactam, 3rd generation cephalosporins, ertapenem
Recent antibiotic treatment: Amoxicillin/clavulanate, fluoroquinolones, trimethoprim/ sulfamethoxazole	Ischemic limb/necrosis/gas forming: Amoxicillin/ clavulanate, piperacillin/ tazobactam, carbapenems, 2nd or 3rd generation cephalosporins + clindamycin or metronidazole
National University Hospital, Singapore (2019)[5]	Cellulitis: Cefazolin or cloxacillin	Septic arthritis/osteomyelitis: IV cefazolin or cloxacillin
	Ulcers: Amoxicillin/clavulanate	Necrotising fasciitis: IV benzylpenicillin + IV ceftazidime + IV clindamycin
		Systemic infection: IV piptazo

Table 5:   Summary of Recommended Antibiotics for MRSA Infections

	Mild Infections	Moderate to Severe Infections
IDSA Guidelines (2012)[2]	Doxycycline Trimethoprim/sulfamethoxazole	Vancomycin Linezolid Daptomycin
IWGDF Guidelines (2020)[4]	Linezolid Trimethoprim/sulfamethoxazole Doxycycline Macrolides	Linezolid Daptomycin Fusidic acid Doxycycline

Culture results should be traced to confirm the causative pathogen so that the appropriate antibiotic regimen can be selected (Tables 4 and 5). Antibiotics can be prescribed for a duration of 1–2 weeks. The patient should be reviewed within the first week after initiation of antibiotics to assess response.

Duration of Antibiotics

Antibiotics should be prescribed for a duration of 1–2 weeks for mild diabetic foot infections. The patient should be reviewed within the first week after initiation of antibiotics to assess response and trace the wound culture results.

Antibiotic treatment can be extended for up to 3–4 weeks in cases where wound infection is improving but is extensive and taking longer than expected to resolve. Extended antibiotic therapy can also be considered for patients with severe peripheral vascular disease.

Patients with osteomyelitis, upon admission to the hospital, generally require surgical resection of the infected bone. Patients who have residual infected bone will require prolonged antibiotics for 6 weeks after the surgery is performed. Antibiotics can be administered parenterally or orally if the pathogen is sensitive to highly bioavailable antibiotics.

Indications for Hospitalisation

Patients with moderate infections extending to deeper structures such as large abscesses, wet gangrene, deep ulcers, septic arthritis, or osteomyelitis will also require admission for surgical intervention. Surgical emergencies like necrotising fasciitis, compartment syndrome, or critical limb ischemia should also be urgently referred for hospitalisation and surgical management.

All patients with severe diabetic foot infections should be admitted to a tertiary institution for closer monitoring and intravenous antibiotics. Hemodynamically unstable patients should immediately be referred to the emergency department, as they may require fluid resuscitation and urgent blood investigations to evaluate for metabolic and cardiovascular derangements.

Hospitalisation may also be considered in the following groups of patients with mild to moderate infections:

- Patients with poorly controlled diabetes and severe hyperglycemia.
- Patients with comorbidities like peripheral vascular disease, renal failure, or immunocompromised states that may impede wound healing.
- Patients with complex social set-ups and poor home support.

- Patients with psychological vulnerabilities that may affect their ability to care for their wounds.
- Patients who fail outpatient management.

References

1. A. Nather, S.B. Chionh, Y.H. Chan, L.J. Chew, C.B. Lin, S.H. Neo, and E.Y. Sim, Epidemiology of diabetic foot problems and predictive factors for limb loss, *J Diabetes Complications* **22**: 77–82 (2008).
2. B.A. Lipsky, A.R. Berendt, P.B. Cornia, J.C. Pile, E.J.G. Peters, D.G. Armstrong, H.G. Deery, J.M. Embil, W.S. Joseph, A.W. Karchmer, M.S. Pinzur, and E. Senneville, 2012 Infectious Diseases Society of America clinical practice guideline for the diagnosis and treatment of diabetic foot infections. *Clin Infect Dis* **2012**: 54 (2012).
3. Z. Aziz, K.L. Wong, A. Nather, and C.Y. Huak, Predictive factors for lower extremity amputations in diabetic foot infections, *Diabet Foot Ankle* **2**: 74463 (2011).
4. — *Guidelines on Prevention and Management of Diabetic Foot Disease 2020*, International Working Group on the Diabetic Foot, International Diabetes Foundation, Brussels.
5. *National University Hospital Antibiotics Guidelines 2019.*

Section 5

Dressing Diabetic Foot Wounds

Chapter 13

Choosing the Appropriate Wound Dressing: A Practical Guide

Aziz Nather

Introduction

In dressing a wound to heal, it is important to first understand the basic science of wound healing. The type of dressing to be chosen and the frequency it has to be changed depend on the phase of wound healing the wound is in.

Basic Science of Wound Healing

There are three phases of wound healing (Figure 1):

Inflammatory Phase

This is the first phase — 1–7 days. It is the cleansing phase to remove bacteria. The main cells involved are platelets, neutrophils, and macrophages. The platelets present release several cytokines.

Proliferative Phase

This is the phase of mesenchymal cell proliferation and synthesis of matrix. Angiogenesis occurs with the formation of granulation tissue with

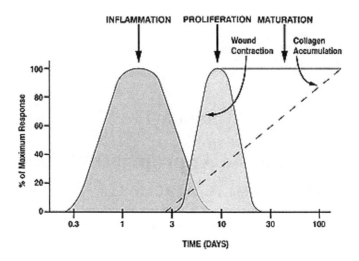

Figure 1:   Phases of Wound Healing

collagen, extracellular matrix, and blood vessels. Main cells involved include fibroblasts, myofibroblasts, and vascular endothelial cells.

Maturation Phase

This is the final phase — day 21 to 1 year. The initial haphazard collagen is degraded and replaced by re-synthesised collagen matrix. Wound remodelling continues up to 1 year.

Take Home Message

- Wounds in the inflammatory phase produce heavy exudates. The dressing may need to be changed daily.
- In the proliferative phase, there is less exudate. The wound may be dressed every other day.
- When a dressing gets soaked, it is time to change the dressing. Often, the patient can tell you how soon the dressing gets soaked and suggest to you how frequently it needs to be changed. This input serves as a useful guide.

Functions of a Dressing

- Protect the wound from trauma and microbial contamination.
- Reduce pain.
- Maintain temperature and moisture of the wound.
- Absorb drainage and debride the wound.
- Control and prevent haemorrhage.
- Provide psychological comfort.

Characteristics of An Ideal Dressing

- Able to remove excess exudate.
- Be waterproof.
- Able to maintain moist wound-healing environment.
- Protect against trauma.
- Allow gaseous exchange.
- Be non-adherent.
- Provide barrier to pathogens.
- Be safe and easy to use.
- Provide thermal insulation.

Types of Wound Dressings

There are various types of wound dressings. Table 1 describes the characteristics of the wound and the recommended category of dressing to be used.

Table 1:   Choice of Wound Dressing to be used

Characteristics of Wound	Recommended Category of Dressing to Use
• Low exudate	Hydrocolloid, hydrofibre (Figure 2)
• Dry necrotic wound	Hydrogel
• Moderate exudate	Alginate
• Moderate to heavy exudate	Foam (Figure 3)
• Infected wound	Antimicrobial (Figure 4)
	○ Silver dressing
	○ Iodine dressing

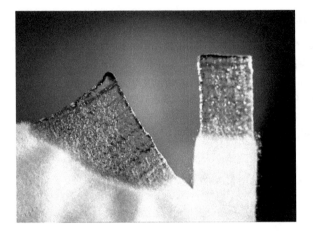

Figure 2:   Hydrofibre Dressing

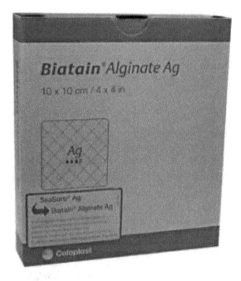

Figure 3:   Foam Dressing

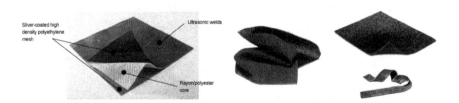

Figure 4:   Antimicrobial Dressings Containing Silver

Summary

Selection of the appropriate dressing is critical for optimal wound healing. Wound dressing is an important adjunct to wound treatment. However, treating the underlying problem is still the most essential part of wound treatment to achieve good wound healing.

Chapter 14

Dressing A Wound: A Step-by-Step Guide for the General Practitioner

Aziz Nather, Michelle Lee Jia Hui, and Tan Chin Fen

Introduction

In dressing a wound, it is important to choose the appropriate dressing to be used. It is also important to decide on how frequently the dressing needs to be changed. The latter depends on the amount of exudate the wound produces and the type of wound being treated — infected wound, ischaemic wound, etc.

Components of a Wound Dressing

There are two components:

- cleansing solution,
- wound product.

Cleansing Solution

Choose a cleansing solution:

- ***Normal Saline 0.9%***
  For a clean wound, use normal saline (Figure 1(a)). This is available in vials or bottles. Normal saline in 1 L bottle once opened must be discarded within 24 hours.
    It is isotonic and safe to use.
    It is cheap.
    It is available in vials or bottles.
- ***Chlorhexidine Gluconate 0.05%***
  For a dirty wound, it may be preferable to use chlorhexidine gluconate (Figure 1(b)).
- ***Acetic Acid 0.25%***
  For wounds infected by *Pseudomonas aeruginosa*, acetic acid 0.25% is the preferred cleansing solution.

Wound Product

Choose the appropriate wound product for each type of wound (Figure 2a,b).

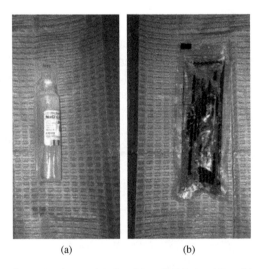

(a)   (b)

Figure 1:   Normal Saline (a) and Chlorhexidine (b).

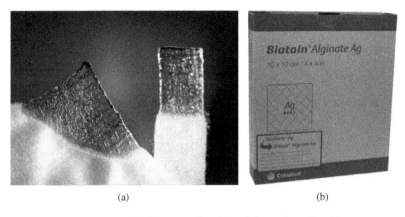

(a)   (b)

Figure 2:   Hydrofibre Dressing (a) and Foam Dressing (b).

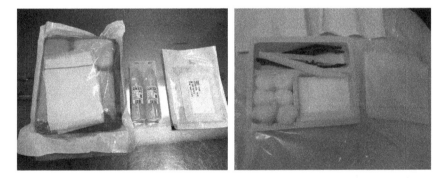

Figure 3:   Disposable Dressing Set

- *Hydrofibre dressing* is used for a low exudate wound.
- *Foam dressing* can be used for a medium exudate wound. It can absorb a large amount of exudate.

Disposable Dressing Set

This basic dressing kit contains the following items (Figure 3):

- Normal saline 0.9% 2 vials (20 mL each)
- Plastic drape
- Paper towel
- Waste bag

- Cotton balls
- Gauze
- Forceps × 3

Procedure

- ***Step 1 — Take a bath before dressing***
- Cover the wound with the plastic bag.
- Take a bath.

- ***Step 2 — Open soiled dressing***
- Wash hands thoroughly.
- Wear gloves (non-sterile).
- Remove soiled dressing and discard it into waste bin.
- Measure the *length* and *width* of the wound using a *disposable paper ruler* (Figure 4a,b).
- Measure the *depth* of the wound using a *swab stick*.
- Wash hands.

- ***Step 3 — Prepare dressing set using aseptic technique***
- Check *expiry date* of dressing set, cleansing solution, and wound product selected.
- Wash hands.
- *Pour chlorhexidine solution* into empty compartment of tray (Figure 5a).

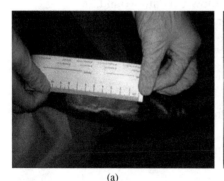
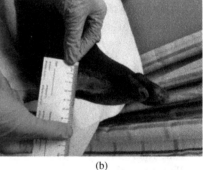

(a)   (b)

Figure 4:   Measuring Length (a) and Width (b) of Wound

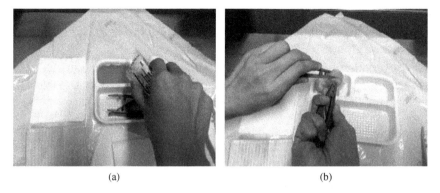

(a)   (b)

Figure 5:   Preparing Dressing Set

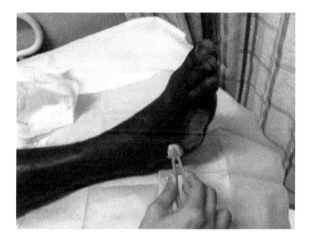

Figure 6:   Cleaning Wound with Chlorhexidine

- *Soak cotton balls* in solution and squeeze dry using *two clean Forceps* (Figure 5b).
- Put them into the next empty compartment of tray.

- ***Step 4 — Cleansing of Wound***
- Pick one prepared cotton ball with a *forceps* (*blue*) and transfer to another *forceps* (*yellow*).
- Use *pink forceps* to *clean the wound* (Figure 6).
- Use *blue forceps* to pick further cotton balls from tray.
- Clean *inside of the wound* first and discard used cotton balls into the yellow plastic bag.
- Use other cotton balls to clean the *surrounding skin*.

- ***Step 5 — Dabbing the wound dry***
- Use a gauze with *normal saline* to clean the inside of the wound to remove all traces of chlorhexidine.
- Use another gauze with saline to clean the surrounding skin.
- Finally, pick one gauze to *dab the inside of the wound* and discard (Figure 7).
- Use another gauze to *dab the surrounding skin.*

- ***Step 6 — Applying the wound product***
- *Cut wound product to required size and shape.*
- Use two clean forceps (first blue forceps and the third forceps in the tray) to pick up the wound product.
- *Apply wound product* onto the wound (Figure 8).

- ***Step 7 — Secure wound product***
- Apply foam.
- *Secure with micropore tape* (Figure 9a).
- *Apply crepe bandage* (Figure 9b).

- ***Step 8 — Give prescription and follow-up date***
  Prescribe the following before sending the patient home:

- cleansing solution,
- wound product
  in sufficient amount for dressing the wound till the next follow-up.

Give the next follow-up date for 1, 2, or 4 weeks later.

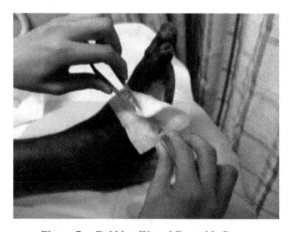

Figure 7:   Dabbing Wound Dry with Gauze

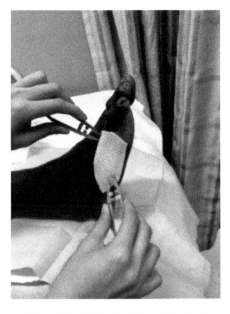

Figure 8: Applying Wound Product

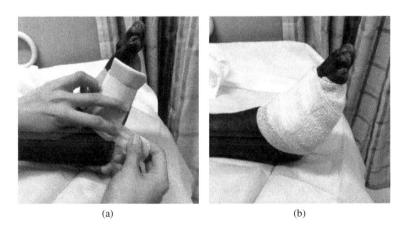

(a)   (b)

Figure 9: Securing Wound Product (a) and Applying Crepe Bandage (b)

- ***Step 9 — Education on wound care***
- Educate the patient on wound care using a *brochure*.
- Teach the patient on *signs of wound infection* (Figure 10).

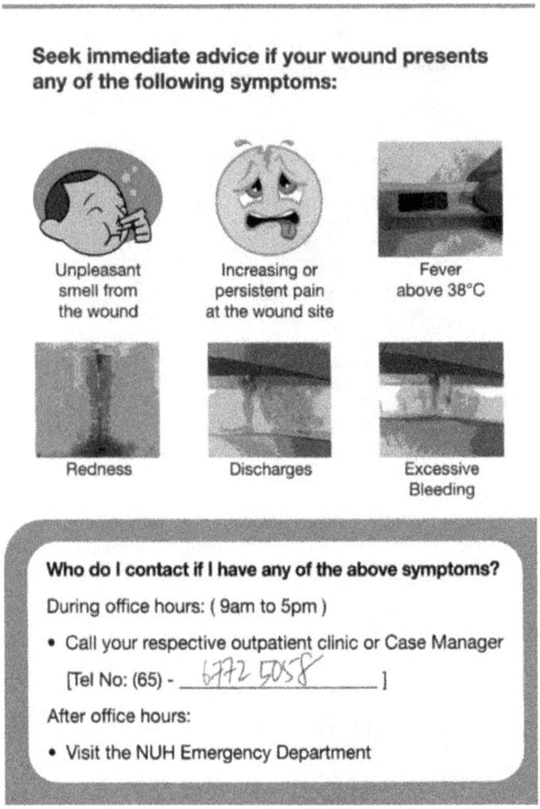

Figure 10:   Signs of Wound Infection

Advise the patient to return to the clinic if the wound presents with one of the following symptoms:

- *unpleasant smell* from wound,
- increasing or persistent *pain* at wound site,
- *fever* more than 38 degrees,
- *redness of wound*,
- *pus discharging from wound*,
- *excessive bleeding* from wound,
- *dressing soaked* before time (too much exudate).

Give the patient your cl*inic contact number.*

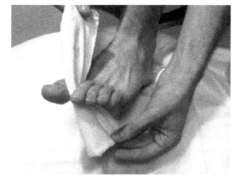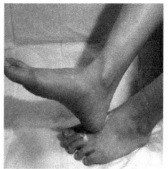

(a) Dry between the toes to prevent maceration

(b) Use your other foot to help with applying cream if you are unable to reach

Figure 11:   Care of Foot

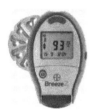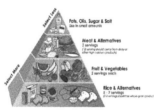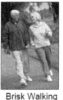

Brisk Walking   Indoors stationary cycling

Figure 12:   Education on Diabetes

- *Step 10 — Educate on foot care*
  Educate the patient on care of the foot:

- Keep foot clean and dry (Figure 11a).
- Use moisturiser to prevent dry skin (Figure 11b).

- *Step 11 — Educate patient on diabetes*
- Must control diabetes (Figure 12).
- Take medication regularly.
- Monitor diabetes regularly using glucometer (Figure 12).
- Follow diabetic diet (Figure 12).
- Exercise regularly (Figure 12).

Section 6

Managing Patients with Diabetic Foot Wounds

Chapter 15

Getting to Know the Operation Performed on Your Patient

Aziz Nather

Introduction

Many of your patients seen in your clinic may have an operation or an amputation performed. Once the wound has healed, and the patient discharged from the hospital outpatient clinic, the patient may be sent back to you for regular follow-ups and long-term care. It is therefore important that as the family practitioner, you should understand a little about the operation that has been performed.

Surgical Debridement

Debridement — excision of necrotic, devitalised, or infected tissue — is the commonest operation performed on diabetic foot. It plays a very important role in the management of diabetic foot wounds[1] (Figure 1). If it is properly performed, it leaves a healthy and vascularised tissue to promote wound healing (Figure 2).

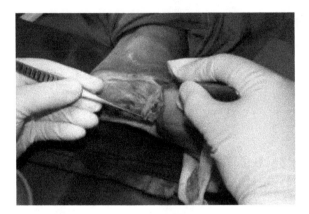

Figure 1:   Excision of Infected and Devitalised Tissue in Sole of Foot

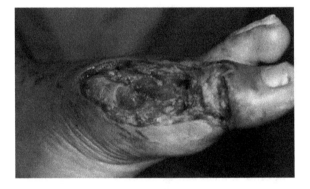

Figure 2:   After Excision of Infected Tissue on Dorsum of Foot

Split Skin Grafting

After debridement, smaller wounds are left to heal on their own. Larger wounds may need split skin grafting. In this procedure, donor skin is taken from the thigh in the normal leg using a dermatome (Figures 3 and 4).

The donor skin is then applied to the recipient wound and stitched in place. A flavine wool dressing is then applied (Figures 5 and 6).

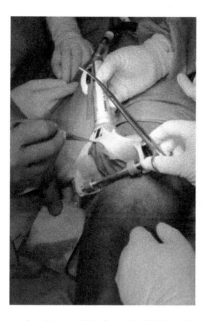

Figure 3: Procuring Donor Skin from the Thigh with a Dermatome

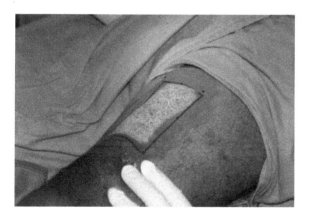

Figure 4: Donor Site After Procurement of Skin

Minor Amputations

In several patients, debridement alone may not suffice. An amputation is also needed to clear the infection. Whenever possible, a minor or distal amputation[1,2] is performed (Table 1) in order to achieve limb salvage.

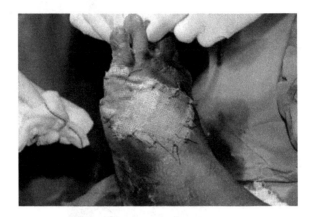

Figure 5:   Stitching Skin Graft in Place in Wound on Dorsum of Foot

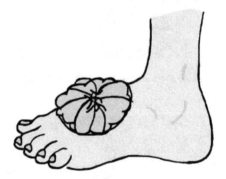

Figure 6:   Applying Flavine Wool Dressing to Keep Graft in Good Position

Classification on Amputations

Ray Amputation

The smallest and commonest amputation performed is the ray amputation — an amputation through the metatarsal bone (Figures 7–9).

In some cases, disarticulation of the toe is done at the metatarsophalangeal joint, if the infection does not extend to the web space.

Trans-Metatarsal Amputation

If more than one ray is involved and the distal part of the forefoot is compromised, a trans-metatarsal amputation is performed[1] (Figures 10 and 11). For this to heal successfully, the dorsalis pedis pulse must be palpable and there is good perfusion in the forefoot — ankle-brachial index >0.7.[1,2]

Table 1: Nather's Classification on Amputation

Amputation Level	Minor (Distal) Amputation (Limb Salvage Achieved)	Major (Proximal) Amputation (Limb Lost)
Fore-foot	Toe disarticulation	
	Ray amputation	
	Trans-metatarsal	
Mid-foot	Lisfranc	
	Chopart	
Hindfoot	Syme	
	Pirogoff	
Trans-tibial		Below knee
Through-the-knee		Through knee
Trans-femoral		Above knee
Hip		Disarticulation

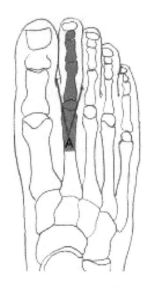

Figure 7: Diagrammatic Representation of Second Ray To Be Excised

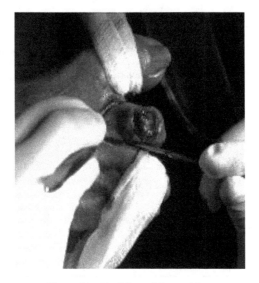

Figure 8:   Excision of Second Ray

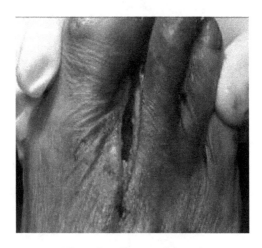

Figure 9:   Closure of wound

Mid-foot Amputations

Lisfranc amputation[1] at level of tarsometatarsal joints (Figure 12) and Chopart amputation[1] at level of Chopart joint: talonavicular joint and calcaneocuboid joints.[1]

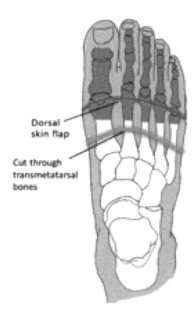

Dorsal skin flap

Cut through transmetatarsal bones

Figure 10:   Curvilinear Line of Osteotomy of All Five Metatarsal Bones (in Green)

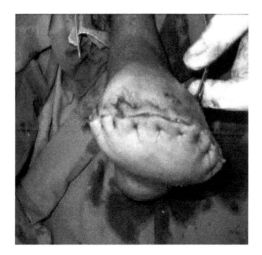

Figure 11:   Wound Closure of Trans-metatarsal Stump

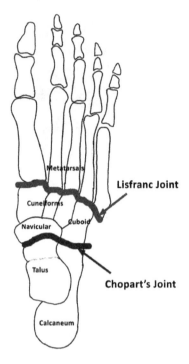

Figure 12:   Lisfranc and Chopart Joints

Pirogoff Amputation

In cases with infection involving both the forefoot and the mid-foot, limb salvage can still be achieved by performing a hindfoot amputation: the Pirogoff amputation[1,2] (see Table 1 and Figures 13–15).

A Pirogoff amputation can only heal successfully if the posterior tibial pulse is palpable and the perfusion in the foot is good — ankle-brachial index >0.7.[1,2]

Why Distal Amputation Preferred

This is because 80% of minor amputees are alive at 2 years compared to only 50% of major amputees being alive at 2 years.[2] Therefore, distal or minor amputation should be performed whenever possible. Also, limb salvage is achieved with this amputation.

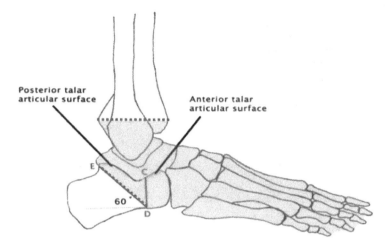

Figure 13:   Osteotomy of Distal Tibia and Mid-calcaneum

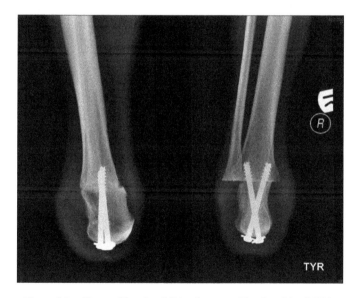

Figure 14:   X-rays Showing Mid-calcaneum Fixed to Distal Tibia

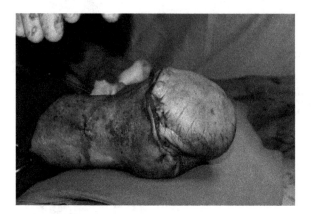

Figure 15:   Closure of Pirogoff Stump

Major Amputations

A major or proximal amputation (Table 1) is only performed when the infection is too far advanced to get away with a distal amputation or when both foot pulses, dorsalis pedis and posterior tibial, are not palpable and the perfusion in the foot is poor.

When a major amputation is performed, limb salvage has failed. The limb is lost and a prosthesis has to be fitted for walking.

Below-knee Amputation

The commonest major amputation performed is the below-knee amputation: the trans-tibial amputation[1] (Table 1, Figures 16 and 17).

Above-knee Amputation

With better care of our diabetic patients today, an above-knee amputation[1] (Figures 18 and 19) is less commonly performed.

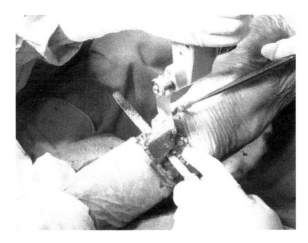

Figure 16: Cutting Tibia with an Oscillating Saw

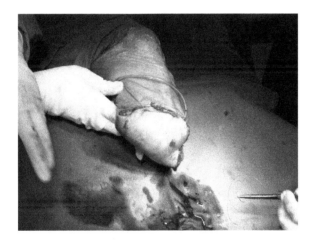

Figure 17: Closure of Below-knee Stump

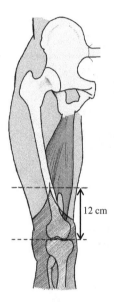

12 cm

Figure 18:   Amputation Level of Above-knee Amputation

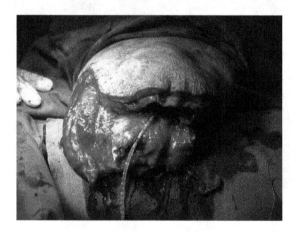

Figure 19:   Closure of Above-knee Stump

References

1. A. Nather (ed.), *Surgery for Diabetic Foot. A Practical Operative Manual*, World Scientific Publishing Co Pte Ltd, New Jersey, London, Singapore, Taipei, Tokyo (2016).
2. A. Nather and K.L. Wong, Distal amputations for the diabetic foot, *Diabetic Foot Ankle.* **4**: 21288 (2013).

Chapter 16

When to Refer Diabetic Foot Complications?

Aziz Nather and Amaris Lim Shu Min

Introduction

With diabetes becoming increasingly prevalent in Singapore, it is crucial to monitor for and detect complications of diabetes. While some complications of diabetes can be managed in primary care, certain diabetic foot complications require further evaluation and treatment that may not easily be available in the primary care setting.

Which diabetic foot complications would then require referral to specialists? And how urgently should they be reviewed by specialists?

This chapter aims to briefly cover the indications for referral for various diabetic foot complications that may present to the clinic or be picked up on diabetic foot screening.

Performing Diabetic Foot Screening

The Ministry of Health (MOH) recommends yearly screening for cardiovascular risk factors, diabetic nephropathy, and eye screening for diabetic retinopathy.

Similarly, MOH also recommends that all patients with newly diagnosed diabetes should undergo diabetic foot screening,[1] followed by a yearly foot examination subsequently.

In Singapore, podiatrists are few in number. They do not conduct yearly foot screening for patients diagnosed with diabetes. A few trained assistant nurses in diabetes clinics in hospitals perform this function. General practitioners can also play an important role in performing this foot screening for their own patients with newly diagnosed diabetes and subsequently yearly foot examination.

What is Diabetic Foot Screening?

The aim of foot screening is to detect early the "foot at risk" — one with the potential to ulcerate. The four risk signs[2] are as follows:

- loss of protective sensation,
- absence of one or both foot pulses,
- presence of foot deformity or callosity,
- inability to reach foot or visual impairment.

History

A detailed history should be taken to include the following:

- Medical History
  - o date diabetes diagnosed,
  - o current treatment for diabetes,
  - o lifestyle.
- History of Foot Conditions
  - o presence of "pins and needles",
  - o previous wound/amputation,
  - o footwear used outdoors.

Examination

- General Patient Examination: Look for
  - o cataract,
  - o conjunctival pallor,
  - o sallow appearance,
  - o dehydration.

- Vital Signs
  - pulse rate,
  - respiratory rate,
  - blood pressure.
- General Foot Assessment: Look for
  - foot deformity,
  - previous amputation,
  - wound,
  - callosity,
  - fungal infection,
  - ingrown toenail,
  - trophic skin changes: shiny skin, loss of hair, pallor, hyperpigmentation, trophic nail changes.
- Vascular Assessment
  - colour and temperature of skin,
  - pulp capillary refill (prolonged if >2 seconds),
  - dorsalis pedis pulse,
  - posterior tibial pulse.
- Assessment for Sensory Neuropathy
  - Pinprick sensation
    Depth of Neuropathy
    - Mild: hyperaesthesia/paraesthesia
    - Moderate: hypoaesthesia
    - Severe: anaesthesia
    Extent of Neuropathy
    - Mild: up to midfoot
    - Moderate: up to ankle
    - Severe: up to mid-shin or beyond
  - Position sense (proprioception)
    Loss of position sense is characteristic of Charcot joint disease
  - Vibration sense
    Assess by placing 128 Hz tuning fork over bony points of the foot — first metatarsal head, malleoli, and tibia

Referring Abnormal Findings of Diabetic Foot Screening

Table 1 indicates who you need to refer to when you find any abnormal finding of the diabetic foot screening.

Table 1:   Who to Refer to for an Abnormal Finding of Diabetic Foot Screening

Abnormal Findings on General Examination	
Callosities	Refer podiatry (routine)
	Educate on foot care and footwear
Foot deformities	Refer to orthopaedic surgery (routine)
Skin tears and wounds	Monitor closely for signs of infection or poor healing
	Look for evidence of vasculopathy or neuropathy
Trophic skin changes without wounds	Continue regular diabetic foot screening
	Look for evidence of vasculopathy or neuropathy
Abnormal Findings on Vascular and Neurologic Assessment	
1 or both pulses not palpable 1 or both pulses poorly felt	Refer to vascular surgery (routine)
Cool foot, prolonged capillary refill time (>2 seconds)	Refer to vascular surgery (routine)
Signs of critical limb ischemia (rest pain, gangrene, non-healing wounds)	Refer to emergency department
Any neuropathy	Refer to endocrinologist (routine)

These patients require more detailed evaluation in a specialist clinic to determine which patients require further management. Early intervention in such cases is the key to prevent the development of a foot "at risk" into becoming a full diabetic foot complication.

Patient Education

Complete the foot screening process by providing patient education on the following:

- *Care of Diabetes*
  o   regular medication
  o   regular monitoring
  o   healthy, balanced diet
  o   exercise
  o   no smoking/alcohol

- ***Care of the Foot***
    - o   foot hygiene
    - o   skin care
    - o   nail care
          inspect your own foot daily
- ***Choice of Footwear***
    - o   *what are appropriate shoes*
    - o   *what are inappropriate shoes*
    - o   *advice to wear shoes outdoors*

Referring Diabetic Foot Complications that Present to Your Clinic

Some patients may have diabetic foot complications that develop in between their annual foot screening. These patients may present acutely to the clinic. Table 2 provides a guide of who to refer to for the diabetic foot complication found.

Table 2:   Guide to Refer Diabetic Foot Complication Presenting in Your Clinic

Charcot joint disease	Refer to orthopaedic surgery clinic (routine)
Poorly healing ulcer (no signs of infection)	Refer to orthopaedic surgery clinic (early)
Dry gangrene	Refer to vascular surgery clinic (early)
Wet gangrene	Refer to emergency department
Abscess of foot	Refer to emergency department
Poorly healing ulcer (with signs of infection)	Refer to emergency department
Moderate/severe cellulitis	Rule out necrotising fasciitis
+/– SIRS	Refer to emergency department for closer monitoring and IV antibiotics
Osteomyelitis	Refer to emergency department
Septic arthritis	Refer to emergency department urgently • will require surgery for joint aspiration and washout
Necrotising Fasciitis	Refer to emergency department urgently • call an ambulance if possible • will require IV antibiotics and surgery urgently

(Continued)

Table 2   (*Continued*)

Patient with foot infection and systemically unwell	Refer to emergency department urgently
≥2 of the following:	• patient may deteriorate rapidly and will require close monitoring and IV antibiotics
• temperature >38°C or <36°C	
• heart rate >90 beats/ min	
• respiratory rate >20 breaths/min or $PaCO_2$ <32 mmHg	
• white blood cell count >12 000 or <4000 cells/µL or ≥10% immature (band) forms	

References

1. *Clinical Practice Guidelines for Managing Diabetes Mellitus*, Ministry of Health, Singapore (2006).
2. G.P. Leese *et al.*, Stratification of foot ulcer risk in patients with diabetes: a population-based study, *Int J Clin Pract.* **60**(5): 541–545 (2006).

Section 7

Educating Patients with Diabetic Foot Wounds

Chapter 17

Living with Diabetes

Aziz Nather, Eda Lim Qiao Yan and Mae Chua Chui Wei

What is Diabetes?

Causes

The cause of diabetes is usually due to high blood glucose levels as a result of ineffectiveness of insulin. Insulin is the hormone that causes cells to take up glucose from blood.

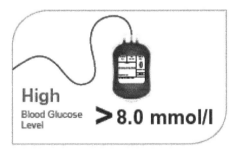

Symptoms

There are four tell-tale signs of diabetes:

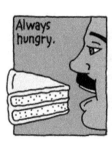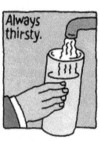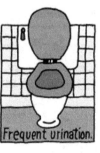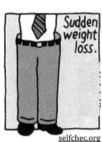

selfchec.org

Complications

Diabetes leads to other health problems. It can result in disability or in more severe cases, death. Such disabilities include the following:

- blindness,
- stroke,
- kidney disease,
- heart attack,
- diabetic foot problems.

Diagnosis

The best way of determining if you have diabetes is to perform a blood glucose test.

	Fasting Blood Glucose
Normal	6.0 mmol/L and below
Pre-diabetes	6.6–6.9 mmol/L
Diabetes	7.0 mmol/L and above

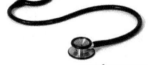

www.ferno.com.au

Treatment: Medication

Insulin Injections — Type 1 Diabetes

Insulin injections help regulate blood glucose levels. Insulin is injected into the layer of fat under the skin.

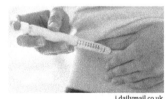

i.dailymail.co.uk

Avoid injecting the same spot each time as this leads to dents or swelling of skin.

Oral Tablets — Type 2 Diabetes

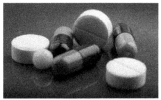

Oral tablets contain hypoglycaemic agents that stimulate the pancreas to release insulin and make body tissues more sensitive to insulin. You must follow through with your course of medication.

static1.squarespace.com

Be sure to administer the injection or take oral tablets ON TIME!

Monitoring

Regular monitoring of one's diabetes is important to prevent diabetic complications. As a patient with diabetes, you should undergo the following:

✓ Hypocount self-monitoring
✓ HbA1c test
✓ Annual eye examination
✓ Annual foot examination

Hypocount Self-monitoring

You should get a glucometer to monitor your blood glucose level closely at home. Follow the following steps:

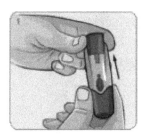
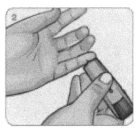
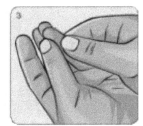

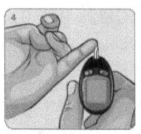 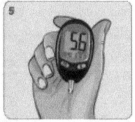 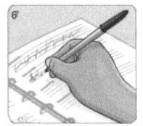

abbottdiabetescare.co.uk

Frequency of self-monitoring:

Treatment Type	Frequency
Insulin	2–3 times a day, 2–3 days weekly
Non-insulin	

Recommended timings for testing:

Morning	Afternoon	Night
Before breakfast	Before lunch	Before dinner
1–2 hours after breakfast	1–2 hours after lunch	1–2 hours after dinner
		Before bed

Reading your glucometer:

Time	Glucometer Reading (mmol/L)		
	Good	Acceptable	Poor
Before meal	6.1–8.0	8.1–10.0	>10.0
After meal	7.1–10.0	10.1–13.0	>13.0

Hypoglycaemia — Too Low Blood Sugar Levels (<3.9 mmol/L)

Symptoms

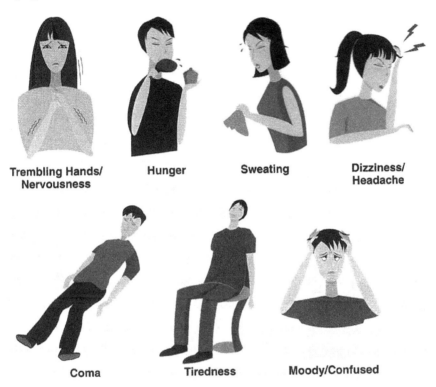

Trembling Hands/   Hunger   Sweating   Dizziness/
Nervousness   Headache

Coma   Tiredness   Moody/Confused

What you should do:

- Check your blood sugar level (it is low if it is <3.9 mmol/L).
- Take your meal or snack immediately if it is already planned for within the next 30 minutes; otherwise.
- Take some sugar (15 g) = 120 mL of regular Coke or three glucose tabs.
- Check your blood sugar level again in 15 minutes.

Hyperglycaemia — Too High Blood Sugar Levels (>14 mmol/L)

Symptoms

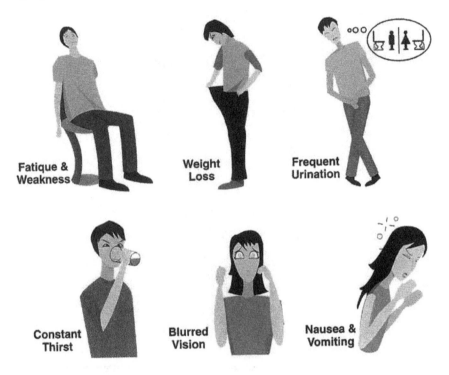

What you should do:

- Check if you are unwell.
- Ensure that you have taken your medication.
- Check your blood sugar level (2–4 hourly) until it is less than 14 mmol/L.
- Check urine ketones.
- Call your doctor or nurse if your/you're
  - blood sugar levels are 14 mmol/L or greater for more than 6 hours,
  - urine ketones are present for more than 6 hours,
  - unable to take fluids or food for 4 hours,
  - severe abdominal pain,
  - still feeling unwell.

HbA1c Test

The test measures how much glucose is attached to your haemoglobin. It reflects an average blood glucose level over a period of 2–3 months. This allows for better control and monitoring of blood glucose levels.

- Frequency: Once every 3 months.
- The acceptable HbA1c level is 6.5–8.0%.

Eye Examination

Visit the hospital/polyclinic for an eye examination every year. This is to treat any early onset of eye problems.

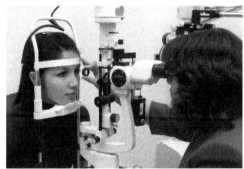

www.cleverdoctors.com

Foot Screening

Visit the hospital/polyclinic for a foot screening every year. This is to treat any diabetic foot problems.

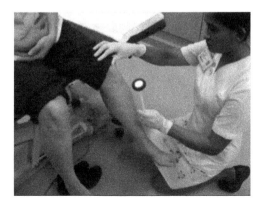

Healthy Lifestyle

Diet

Health Promotion Board, Singapore

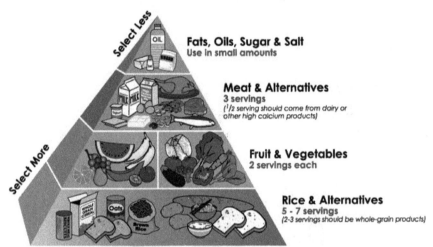

Control your intake of carbohydrates. Maintain a balanced diet by following the healthy diet pyramid that indicates the proportion of different food that you should consume.

Regulate your carbohydrate intake as it significantly affects your blood glucose level. Count your calorie intake for each meal. Do not take more than 1,800 calories a day.

General guidelines on diet
✓ Choose "low fat" or "healthier choice" options.
✓ Use healthier cooking methods, such as broiling, boiling, steaming, baking, stir-frying, or poaching.
✓ Eat on time.
✓ Eat slowly.
✓ Drink eight glasses of water every day.

Health Promotion Board, Singapore

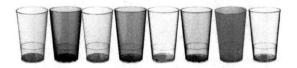

Weight

Excess body fat prevents insulin from working properly. Keep check of your health by calculating your Body Mass Index (BMI) regularly.

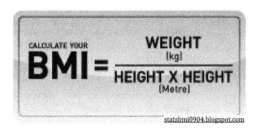

The healthy range is 18.5–22.9 kg/m².

Exercise

Exercise regularly to lower your blood glucose level. Exercise uses up glucose and burns body fat. It also

- improves blood circulation,
- strengthens your heart,
- relieves stress.

How often should you exercise?
30 minutes a day, at least 5 days a week.

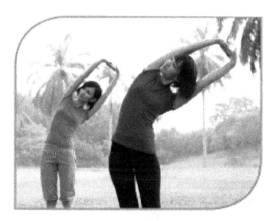

You can break up these 30 minutes into smaller parts and rest in between.

What types of exercises are suitable?

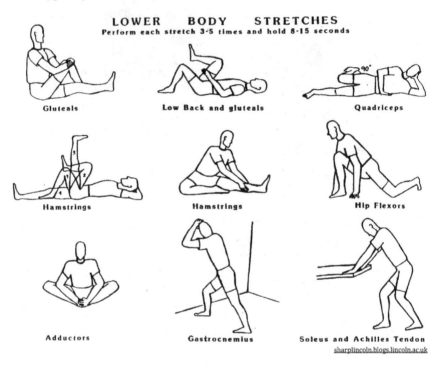

LOWER   BODY   STRETCHES
Perform each stretch 3-5 times and hold 8-15 seconds

Gluteals   Low Back and gluteals   Quadriceps

Hamstrings   Hamstrings   Hip Flexors

Adductors   Gastrocnemius   Soleus and Achilles Tendon

sharplincoln.blogs.lincoln.ac.uk

Other exercises:

- brisk walking,
- climbing stairs,
- indoor stationary cycling,
- low-impact aerobics,
- line dancing,
- swimming.

No Smoking

Smoking accelerates the onset of diabetic complications. It narrows your blood vessels and restricts blood flow.

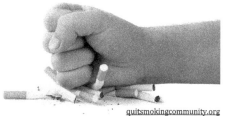

quitsmokingcommunity.org

Tips to help you stop smoking

✓ Do not carry a lighter around with you.
✓ When the urge to smoke hits, take a deep breath. Hold it in for 10 seconds and then release it slowly. Repeat this.
✓ Spend your time freely in places where smoking is prohibited.
✓ Substitute cigarettes with fresh fruit, crunchy vegetables or sugarless gum.
✓ Exercise more.

No Alcohol

Alcohol causes your blood glucose level to rise.

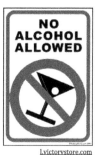

 Drinking limits for diabetics
• Females: 1 drink per day
• Males: 2 drinks per day

*1 drink = 354 mL beer/147 mL wine.

l.victorystore.com

Chapter 18

Taking Care of the Foot

Aziz Nather, Wee Lin and Mae Chua Chui Wei

Introduction

The key to healthy feet is PREVENTION. One must know how to take good care of our feet to prevent foot complications from occurring. This chapter describes five steps one can follow to keep the feet healthy.

Step 1: Foot Hygiene

Proper foot hygiene is the first step to maintaining healthy feet. Bacteria and other harmful micro-organisms accumulate in your feet through their daily use. They need to be removed before they cause harm to your feet.

Keep your feet clean and dry

- Wash your feet with warm water at least twice a day.
- Do not soak for more than 5 minutes.

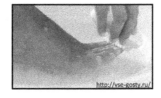

For normal skin, wash with <u>mild soap</u>.

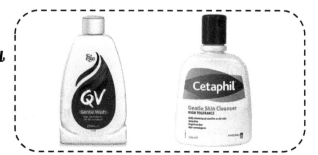

What is mild soap?
- Does not contain artificial fragrance
- Contains ingredients that sooth and refresh the skin

If your feet are <u>dry</u>, do not use soap. Use a <u>gentle skin cleanser</u> instead.

- Dry your feet with a clean towel, especially the web spaces between the toes. If they are not dried properly, it can lead to skin maceration (softening) and breakdown of skin.

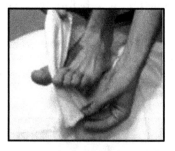

Avoid powdering your feet

- They cause friction and abrasions.
- This causes the skin to break and bacteria to enter the open wound and lead to infection.

AVOID POWDER

Step 2: Skin Care

The skin is the layer that protects your feet from harm. It should be well looked after to keep your feet healthy. Moisturise your feet to prevent dry skin. Keep your skin in top form.

Use moisturiser to prevent dry skin

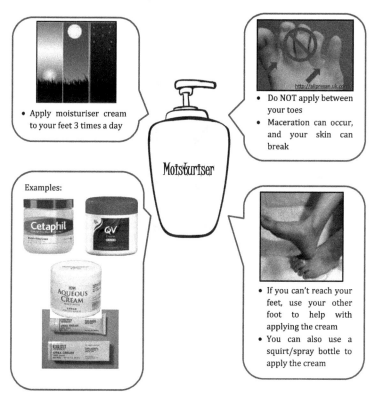

 cut calluses with scissors or nail clipper

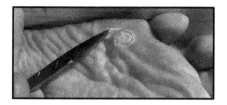

Step 3: Nail Care

Toenails need proper care and attention. Proper nail care ensures no complications from nail problems.

Keep your toenails trimmed

Proper nail care		
• Trim your toenails after showering. They are softer and easier to cut	• Use nail clippers instead of scissors 	• Trim your toenails straight across and not too short • Do not dig into the corners of the nail • Use a nail file to gently file down any sharp corners of the nail 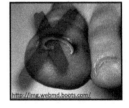

- If you have problems reaching your feet,
  - get a family member/friend to help trim toenails
  - visit a podiatrist for toenail care

Improper Nail Care

- Can result in ingrown toe nail.
- Toenail can break the skin and result in an infection.

http://img.webmd.boots.com/

Step 4: Inspecting Your Feet

Your feet require daily inspection. Any injury sustained will be detected early. This is especially important for diabetic patients. They may have numbness of the feet and are unable to feel pain when injured.

Inspect your feet daily

- Look and feel for any cuts, blisters, abrasions, calluses, etc.
- Yellow toenails that are thick and brittle means you are likely to have a fungal nail infection.

- Look at the
  1. toes,
  2. nails,
  3. web spaces (spaces between toes),
  4. top of foot,
  5. sole of foot,
  6. heel.

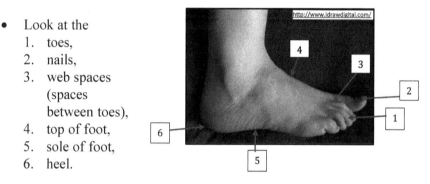

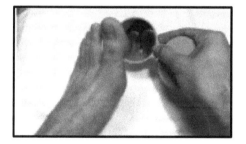

Use mirror to look at bottom of foot or get a family member/friend to help

- Inform a healthcare professional if you find any abnormality.
- Consult a doctor for annual screening of your feet.

Step 5: First Aid for Foot

One must have first aid available in case of any injury. It can mean a huge difference whether the injury recovers quickly or develops into a serious one.

First Aid Kit

- Keep a first aid box that contains the following:
    1. Cleansing solution
    2. Gauze pad
    3. Cotton balls
    4. Forceps
    5. Band-aid
    6. Antiseptic cream
       (*Avoid using harsh antiseptics, like alcohol and iodine, and ask your doctor which are safe for you to use*)
    7. Crepe bandage
    8. Saline solution
    9. Calamine lotion

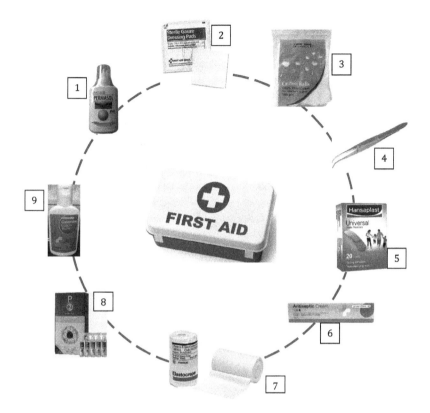

- You can purchase a ready-assembled first aid kit from any major healthcare shop.

Managing Abrasions or Minor Cuts

- Run the injury with clean water, to remove any dirt.
- Use gauze to apply slight pressure on the wound for a few minutes to help stop bleeding.
- Cover the wound with clean dressing. Change the dressing daily.

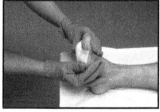

http://www.anklefootmd.com/

- Get medical help if the wound continues to bleed or is caused by rusty objects.

Managing Insect Bites and Stings

- Remove any sting left behind.
- Apply Calamine lotion to soothe the area or an ice pack to reduce swelling.
- Seek medical help if there is increased pain and swelling to counteract possible allergic reaction.

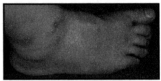

http://www.pattayaunlimited.com/

Managing Bleeding

- For a <u>MINOR</u> wound,
  - o Clean the wound and make sure there are no particles in it.
  - o Press a clean gauze pad over the wound for a few minutes to stop the bleeding.
  - o Apply an antiseptic cream on the surrounding skin and leave to heal.
- <u>HEAVY</u> bleeding,
  - o Call for medical help immediately.
  - o Place a thick pad of bandage over wound and press firmly to control bleeding.
  - o Raise the bleeding part higher than the rest of the body unless there are broken bones.

Managing Burns and Scalds

- <u>Burn:</u> A skin injury caused by direct fire, friction, chemicals, electricity, or radiation.
- <u>Scald:</u> A burn caused by hot liquid or steam.
- Remove all constricting accessories and clothing from the affected area.
- Place under cold running water for at least 10 minutes to ease the pain.
- Avoid breaking any blister that may appear.
- Do NOT apply ointment or other home remedies. They cause further damage or infection.
- Apply aloe vera gel or emergency burn dressings like Burnaid gel or Aluminaid.

- Minor burns can be managed by covering the affected area with sterile gauze, foam, or dressings to minimise pain and to support healing.
- Get medical help immediately if the burn is severe or the area of burn is extensive.

Burnaid gel

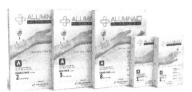

Aluminaid burn dressings

Common Misconceptions

The following represents several misconceptions/myths which diabetic patients may have. However, such myths are in fact false and may cause patients to endanger themselves and their feet. Thus, the following table serves to debunk these myths and instead bring the truth to light.

	Myth	Truth
Myth #1	Calluses are protective and should be left untreated.	Calluses result in increased pressure on the foot. An ulcer may develop.
Myth #2	My foot problems are not serious because they are painless.	Patients with diabetes may have numbness in the feet. They do not feel pain, even when problems develop.
Myth #3	It is alright to test the temperature of water using my feet.	Diabetic patients may have numbness in their feet and will not be able to detect water at high temperatures. The feet may instead develop burns.
Myth #4	Diabetic wounds heal faster than normal.	Diabetic wounds typically heal slower than normal.
Myth #5	A good way to pamper my feet is to soak them in warm water for a long time.	Soaking feet may risk infection if the skin begins to break down. Do not soak for more than 5 minutes.
Myth #6	It is good to treat my feet to some foot reflexology by walking barefoot on the stones at the nearby park.	Diabetic patients may have numbness in their feet and will not be able to detect cuts or injuries sustained by their bare feet. They should not go out of their houses with bare feet.

Summary Tips and Checklist

Here is a checklist for a daily routine to the care of your feet, as well as some summary tips for you to remember.

Checklist for Daily Inspection

☐   Check your feet daily for cuts, blisters, etc.
☐   Use a mirror to see soles of your feet
☐   Always wash feet with soap and water
☐   Remember to wash between the toes
☐   Dry feet carefully using a soft towel
☐   Use moisturiser to keep skin hydrated
☐   Cut toenails straight across
☐   Go for foot screening once a year

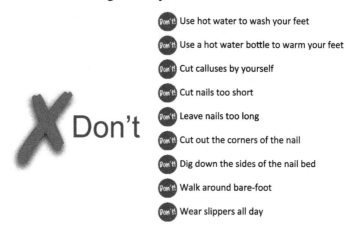

(Don't) Use hot water to wash your feet

(Don't) Use a hot water bottle to warm your feet

(Don't) Cut calluses by yourself

(Don't) Cut nails too short

(Don't) Leave nails too long

(Don't) Cut out the corners of the nail

(Don't) Dig down the sides of the nail bed

(Don't) Walk around bare-foot

(Don't) Wear slippers all day

When Travelling

When we are travelling, there are many other things for us to worry about, such as our luggage, the flight details, and our programme. However, our feet must not be forgotten. Special considerations need to be made to ensure our feet are well taken care of.

Flying to Your Destination

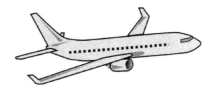

- Constantly sip water to avoid dehydration.
- Wear shoes with adjustable fittings.
- Ask for an aisle seat — walk up and down the aisle every half hour to prevent your feet from swelling.
- Choose a seat with more legroom.

Upon Arrival

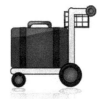

- Be careful of trolleys that may ramp onto your feet
- Arrange for a wheelchair if possible.
- Use a trolley — do not carry heavy luggage.

In Subtropical or Tropical Countries

- Use insect repellent to avoid insect bites.
- Avoid eating, handling, or exposing open wounds to raw seafood in areas where *Vibrio vulnificus* is endemic (bacteria which causes serious damage to the skin).
- Beware of rats which may nibble at your shoes and feet.
- Do not go barefoot when walking on the beach or in the sea.
- Use sun block with high SPF to protect your skin.
- Keep dry skin moisturised.

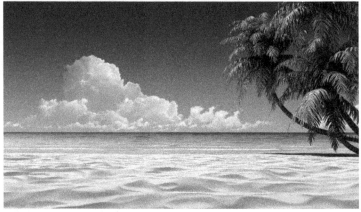

http://pcwallart.com/

Foot Screening

Foot screening is an essential component of caring for your foot. This is to detect the "foot at risk" early for referral to the podiatrist, the orthopaedic surgeon, or the vascular surgeon as early as possible. With foot screening, the rate of foot complications and thereby the amputation rate can both be reduced.

Frequency and Duration

The foot screening should be at least done annually. This is especially important for diabetic patients since wounds may take longer to heal and nerve damage may cause a patient to be insensitive to foot trauma or pain.

Each foot screening takes about 30 minutes to complete.

Where

This can be done at all the hospitals and polyclinics.

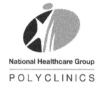

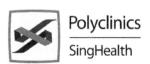

What to Expect: The Procedure

Foot screening includes the taking of the patient's personal and medical history followed by the clinical examination, possibly a neurological assessment as well as a vascular assessment. A simple management plan is also formulated.

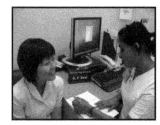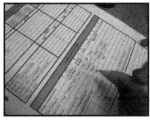

Trained Nurse Taking Down Patient's History

The clinical examination may comprise of the **general foot assessment**, where skin conditions are assessed, the biomechanical assessment, where any foot structure deformities are assessed.

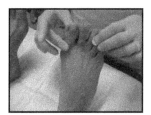

General assessment of the foot

The **neurological assessment** includes five tests which will be performed to assess the neurological condition in the patient's feet.

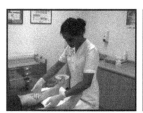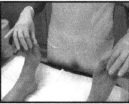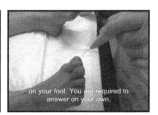

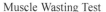

Muscle Wasting Test   Proprioception Test   Monofilament Test

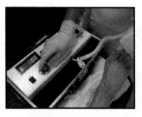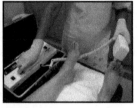

Vibration Perception Test Using Neurothesiometer

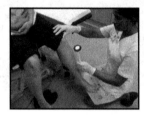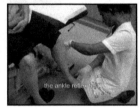

Knee and Ankle Reflex Tests

A **vascular assessment** might also be carried out depending on the hospital or polyclinic.

What to Bring + Wear

- Bring
  - your own footwear,
  - previous insoles,
  - medication for your feet.
- Wear a set of clothes that does not restrict your movements e.g. shorts and t-shirts. Part of your arms and legs may be revealed during the assessment.

Chapter 19

Choosing Your Footwear

Aziz Nather, Zest Ang and Jere Low Wenn

Introduction

As a diabetic, you are at risk of developing foot problems, including foot ulcers. The use of proper footwear is key in protecting yourself against these. It is unfortunate that many diabetics tend to use poor footwear because it is convenient or fashionable, putting their feet in danger of injuries. This chapter will guide you on how to select proper footwear.

What Makes a Good Shoe?

A good shoe will have the following characteristics:

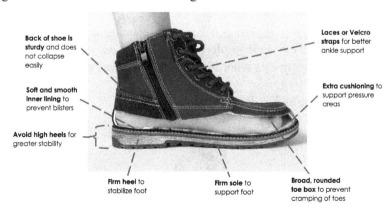

Image Source: http://www.kinderfuesse.com/wie_das_plus12_funktioniert.

175

Shoes made from soft leather are ideal, as are sports shoes and sandals with adjustable straps.

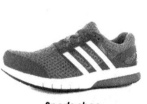 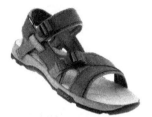

Sports shoe   **Sandal with adjustable straps**

Avoid These!

Poor footwear can cause permanent damage to your feet. These are shoes that you should avoid:

- **Thin-Soled Shoes**

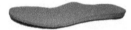

These do not absorb impact well and can cause ulceration and even fractures. Sharp objects can moreover pierce through thin soles easily.
- **High-Heeled Shoes**

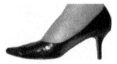

Such shoes result in too much pressure being exerted over your forefeet, which can lead to ulceration. Women are also prone to falls and soft tissue injuries when wearing high-heeled shoes due to poor balance.
- **Shoes with Tight Toe Boxes**

Such shoes can cause toe cramps. The increased friction between your toes may also lead to ulceration.
- **Flip-Flops**

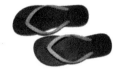

Your toes and heels remain unprotected. The friction between the straps and your toes may also lead to ulceration.

- **Slip-On Shoes**

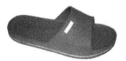

Your feet may move excessively within such shoes, generating a lot of friction, which can lead to foot ulcers.

Choosing Your Shoes — Do's and Don'ts

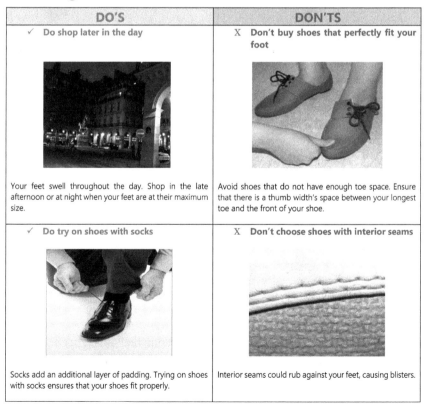

DO'S	DON'TS
✓ Do shop later in the day	X **Don't buy shoes that perfectly fit your foot**
Your feet swell throughout the day. Shop in the late afternoon or at night when your feet are at their maximum size.	Avoid shoes that do not have enough toe space. Ensure that there is a thumb width's space between your longest toe and the front of your shoe.
✓ Do try on shoes with socks	X **Don't choose shoes with interior seams**
Socks add an additional layer of padding. Trying on shoes with socks ensures that your shoes fit properly.	Interior seams could rub against your feet, causing blisters.

(*Continued*)

(Continued)

✓ **Do buy shoes that fit your larger foot**	X **Don't select shoes based on pre-measured shoe sizes**
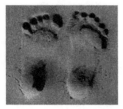	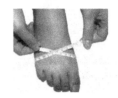
Your feet are of different sizes. Buy shoes that fit your larger foot.	Always try on a new pair of shoes to ensure a proper fit before purchase.
✓ **Do break in new shoes gradually**	X **Don't buy shoes made of plastic or moldable rubber**
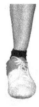	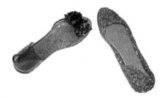
Break in new shoes slowly. Start by wearing your shoes for 30 minutes each day until you are comfortable with them. Check for blisters, cuts and calluses each time.	Avoid shoes made of plastic or non-heatproof, moldable rubber. Leather shoes are good. Shoes made from PVC are acceptable.

Before Wearing Shoes

Always perform the following before wearing your shoes:

- **Wear clean synthetic socks**

Ideal socks: Acrylic, no elastic tops, not too long

Socks provide additional protection for your feet and reduce the risk of blisters and fungal infections. Select socks made of synthetic material, e.g. acrylic, as they are lightweight, durable, and less likely to bunch up. Avoid cotton socks as they tend to trap heat and cause blisters.

You should also avoid knee-high socks and socks with elastic tops.

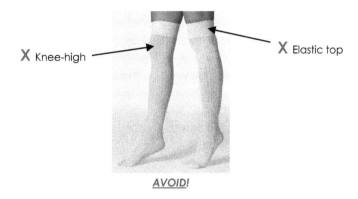

X Knee-high   X Elastic top

AVOID!

Do remember to change your socks daily!

• **Check shoes for damage and foreign bodies**

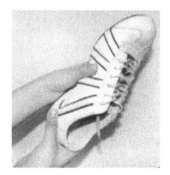

Check both the inside and the outside of your shoes for wear and tear and replace them when they are worn out. Also, shake any foreign bodies, e.g. pebbles or grit, out of your shoes before putting them on.

Fact or Fiction?

The following are a few statements pertaining to the selection and use of footwear. A few are facts while the others are common misconceptions. Can you differentiate fact from fiction?

1. It is alright to go barefoot at home.   True/False
2. We need more than 1 pair of shoes.   True/False
3. I should wear massage slippers regularly as they
    improve blood circulation.   True/False
4. Shoes should fit snugly around the entire foot.   True/False
5. We should never select our shoes based on
    pre-measured shoe sizes.   True/False
6. I should wear tight socks as they will provide
    support for my feet.   True/False

Answers with detailed explanations can be found on the below page.

Answers:

1. **False**

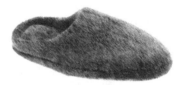

You should wear proper footwear at all times to protect your feet. Ideally, you should wear soft-cushioned slippers when walking around at home.

2. **True**

You should own at least 2 pairs of shoes and alternate between them regularly. This will allow each pair of shoes to air completely before use and prevent each pair from wearing out too quickly.

3. **False**

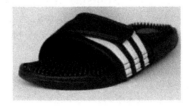

You should avoid wearing massage slippers as they increase pressure over the soles of your feet and can cause foot ulcers.

4. **False**

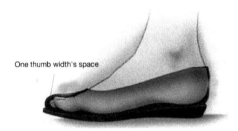

One thumb width's space

A fitting shoe is one where there is a thumb width's space between your longest toe and the front of your shoe. In a poorly fitting shoe, your toes may experience too much friction, which can lead to ulceration.

5. **True**

Always try on a new pair of shoes to ensure a proper fit before purchase. Certain shoes that are marketed as your size may in reality be ill-fitting.

6. **False**

Tight socks should be avoided as they might affect the blood circulation in your feet.

Test Yourself!

How much have you absorbed from this module? Test yourself and find out. Answers can be found on the next page.

Question 1:

Which of the following shoe types is appropriate for daily use by a diabetic patient?

(A) Stilettos
(B) Flip-flops
(C) Sports shoes
(D) Massage slippers

Question 2:
When is the best time to shop for new shoes?

(A) Any time is equally good
(B) In the morning
(C) In the early afternoon
(D) In the evening

Question 3:
_____ socks are the most appropriate for daily wear.

(A) Synthetic-based
(B) Cotton
(C) Wool
(D) Silk

Question 4:
Which of the following statements is **TRUE**?

(A) Online shopping for shoes based on pre-measured shoe sizes is ideal
(B) It is okay to go barefoot at home
(C) I should try on new shoes while wearing socks
(D) I only need one pair of shoes

Question 5:
How often should you change your socks?

(A) Hourly
(B) Daily
(C) Weekly
(D) Monthly

Answers:
(1) C
(2) D
(3) A
(4) C
(5) B

Checklist

Refer to this checklist regularly to refresh your knowledge about proper footwear!

Buying new shoes
- Shop later in the day
- Avoid:
  - High-heeled shoes
  - Slip-on shoes
  - Flip-flops
  - Massage slippers
  - Thin-soled shoes
  - Shoes with interior seams
  - Shoes with tight-toe boxes
  - Shoes made of plastic
  - Shoes made of non-heatproof, moldable rubber
- Try on shoes with socks before purchase
- Buy shoes that fit larger foot
- Ensure a thumb width's space between longest toe and front of shoe
- Break in new shoes gradually

Daily use of footwear
- Alternate between at least two pairs of shoes
- Check shoes for damage and foreign bodies
- Wear clean synthetic socks
- Avoid knee-high socks, socks with elastic tops, and cotton socks

Chapter 20

Education Pamphlets

1. Knowing Diabetes

Aziz Nather and Eda Lim Qiao Yan

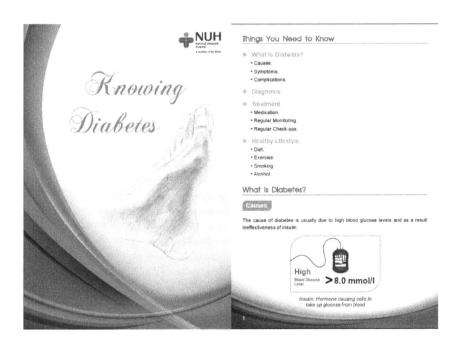

Symptoms

There are **4 tell-tale signs** of diabetes

- ❖ Always thirsty.
- ❖ Sudden weight loss.
- ❖ Frequent urination.
- ❖ Always hungry.

Complications

Diabetes leads to other health problems. It can result in disability or in more severe cases, death.

Excessively high blood glucose causes:

- ❖ Breathlessness.
- ❖ Fatigue.
- ❖ Nausea & Vomiting.
- ❖ Persistent Infections.

Low blood glucose causes:

- ❖ Mental Confusion.
- ❖ Dizziness.
- ❖ Trembling hands.
- ❖ Loss of consciousness.
- ❖ Fatigue.

The long-term effects of low blood glucose are due to the narrowing and hardening of the blood vessels that restricts blood flow and increases their risk of clogging.

Other effects of diabetes can also cause:

- ❖ Blindness.
- ❖ Stroke.
- ❖ Kidney disease.
- ❖ Heart attack.
- ❖ Diabetic foot problems.

Diagnosis

The best way of determining if you have diabetes is to perform a blood glucose test.

	Fasting Blood Glucose
NORMAL	6.0mmol/l and below
PRE-DIABETES	6.6 - 6.9 mmol/l
DIABETES	7.0mmol/l and above

Treatment

Medication

1. Injection of insulin

For Type 1 Diabetes, insulin injections help to regulate blood glucose levels.

Insulin is injected into the layer of fat under the skin. Avoid injecting the same spot each time as this leads to dents or swelling of skin.

2. Oral tablets

For Type 2 Diabetes, take oral tablets (hypoglycaemic agents) prescribed by your doctors and follow through with your course of medication.

> Be sure to administer the injection or take oral tablets ON TIME!

Regular Monitoring

Always monitor your blood glucose level closely.

1. Guidelines:

- ❖ Get a glucometer.
- ❖ Frequency of self-monitoring:

Treatment Type	Frequency
Insulin	2 - 3 times a day, 2 - 3 days weekly
Non-insulin	Frequent enough to achieve glucose targets

- ❖ Recommended timings for testing:

Morning	Afternoon	Night
Before breakfast	Before lunch	Before dinner
1 - 2 hours after breakfast	1 - 2 hours after lunch	1 - 2 hours after dinner
		Before bed

- ❖ Reading your glucometer:

Time	Glucometer Reading (mmol/L)		
	Good	Acceptable	Poor
Before Meal	6.1 - 8.0	8.1 - 10.0	> 10.0
After Meal	7.1 - 10.0	10.1 - 13.0	> 13.0

2. What should I do if I experience low blood glucose symptoms?

- ❖ Fainting Spells.
- ❖ Trembling Hands.
- ❖ Fatigue.

These symptoms typically occur when your blood glucose level is too low (<3.9mmol/l). In such events, eat or drink something sweet.

3. Weight

Keep fit by monitoring your weight regularly. BMI is a reliable indicator of your health.

Keep your BMI in check!

$$BMI = \frac{Weight\ (KG)}{Height^2\ (m^2)}$$

> The healthy range is 18.5 - 22.9 kg/m2

Regular Check-ups

It is important to visit your doctor for the following regular check-ups to keep your health in check.

- ❖ Hemoglobin A1c (HbA1c) test
  - Frequency: Once every 3 months.
  - To monitor your blood glucose level.
  - The acceptable HbA1c level is 6.5 - 8.0%.
- ❖ Eye Check-up
  - Frequency: Annually.
  - To treat any early onset of eye problems.

❖ Foot Examination
  • Frequency: Annually.
  • To treat any Diabetic foot problems.

❖ Urine test
  • Frequency: Annually.
  • To ensure that your kidneys are functioning normally.

Healthy Lifestyle

Diet

Control your intake of carbohydrates. Maintain a balanced diet by following the Healthy Diet Pyramid that indicate the proportion of different food that you should consume.

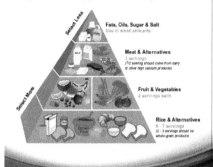

Select Less / Select More

Fats, Oils, Sugar & Salt
Use in small amounts

Meat & Alternatives
3 servings
(1/2 serving should come from dairy or other high calcium products)

Fruit & Vegetables
2 servings each

Rice & Alternatives
5 - 7 servings
(2 - 3 servings should be whole-grain products)

Regulate your carbohydrate intake as it significantly affects your blood glucose level. Count your calorie intake for each meal. Do not take more than 1800 calories a day.

General guidelines on diet

1. Choose 'Low Fat' options.
2. Use healthier cooking methods such as broiling, boiling, steaming, baking, stir-frying or poaching.
3. Eat on time.
4. Eat slowly.
5. Drink 8 glasses of water per day.

Exercise

Exercise regularly to lower your blood glucose level.

Exercise uses up glucose and burns body fat. It also:
  • Improves blood circulation.
  • Strengthens your heart.
  • Relieves stress.

How often should I exercise?

30 minutes a day, at least 5 days a week.

You can break up these 30 minutes into smaller parts and rest in between.

What types of exercises are suitable for me?

Lower Body Stretching

Do each step 3 - 5 times, 8 - 15 seconds each.

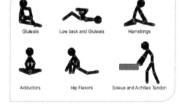

Gluteals / Low back and Gluteals / Hamstrings / Adductors / Hip Flexors / Soleus and Achilles Tendon

Other Exercises

❖ Brisk walking.
❖ Climbing stairs.
❖ Indoor stationary cycling.
❖ Low-impact aerobics.
❖ Line dancing.
❖ Swimming.

Tips for your exercise regime

Pre-Exercise
  • Check your blood glucose twice, 30 minutes apart to ensure that readings are stable.
  • Avoid injecting insulin into limbs that are using for exercise.
  • When exercising in the evening, increase your carbohydrate intake to minimize low blood glucose symptoms.
  • Exercising in the morning, at about 7am, gives optimum health effects.
  • Use a pedometer. Take 10000 steps a day.

During Exercise
  • Carry glucose tablets or sweet drinks in case you experience symptoms of low blood glucose.
  • Always carry an identification tag.
  • Wear well-fitting socks and shoes.
  • Drink plenty of water.
  • Avoid exercising alone.

Post-Exercise
  • Check your blood glucose twice, 30 minutes apart to ensure that readings are stable.
  • Check your feet for redness, cuts or sores.

No Smoking

Smoking accelerates onset of diabetic complications. It narrows your blood vessels and restricts blood flow.

Stop smoking,
or risk your life.

Tips to help you stop smoking

❖ Do not carry a lighter around with you.

❖ When the urge to smoke hits, take a deep breath. Hold it for 10 seconds and then release it slowly. Repeat this.

❖ Spend your free time in places where smoking is prohibited.

❖ Substitute cigarettes with fresh fruits, crunchy vegetables or sugarless gum.

❖ Exercise more.

No Alcohol

Alcohol causes your blood glucose level to rise.

Drinking Limits for diabetics:

❖ Females: 1 drink per day.
❖ Males: 2 drinks per day.

*1 drink = 354 ml beer/ 147 ml wine

10

2. Happy Feet

Aziz Nather and Wee Lin

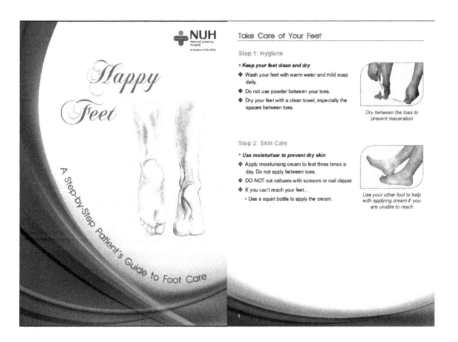

Take Care of Your Feet

Step 1: Hygiene

• Keep your feet clean and dry

❖ Wash your feet with warm water and mild soap daily.

❖ Do not use powder between your toes.

❖ Dry your feet with a clean towel, especially the spaces between toes.

Dry between the toes to prevent maceration

Step 2: Skin Care

• Use moisturiser to prevent dry skin

❖ Apply moisturising cream to feet three times a day. Do not apply between toes.

❖ DO NOT cut calluses with scissors or nail clipper.

❖ If you can't reach your feet...

• Use a squirt bottle to apply the cream.

Use your other foot to help with applying cream if you are unable to reach

Step 3: Nail Care

* **Keep your toenails trimmed**
❖ Trim your toenails after showering.
❖ Use nail clippers.
❖ Trim your toenails straight across.
❖ Use a nail file to file sharp corners.
❖ Do not dig into the corners of the nail.

Trim toenails straight across and not down the corners

Infected Ingrown toenail

Step 4: All About First Aid

❖ Keep a first aid box that contains:
• Cleansing solution.
• Gauze.
• Cotton balls.
• Forceps.
• Antiseptic cream.
• Band-aid.
❖ Clean your wound with the cleansing solution.
❖ Apply the dressing.
❖ Look out for pain, redness, warmth, swelling or discharge.
❖ See a doctor if any sign of pain, redness, swelling or discharge appears.

Step 5: Importance of Foot Inspection

* **Inspect your feet daily**
❖ Inspect your feet carefully including the toes, toenails and web spaces.
❖ Use a mirror to see the bottom of your feet.
❖ Look and feel for cuts, blisters, abrasions, corns, calluses and changes in colour.
❖ Consult a doctor to have your feet screened annually.
❖ Get a family member/ friend to help if you are unable to reach your feet.

Use a mirror to look at the bottom of the foot

Check spaces between toes

Warning!

Telling signs that your foot may be in trouble

❖ Pain in the foot.
❖ Redness or discolouration.
❖ Foot feels hot.
❖ Foot emits a foul smell or odour.
❖ Your Foot has ulcers or blisters.

Debunking Common Misconceptions About Foot Care

	Myth	Truth
Myth #1	Calluses are protective, and should be left untreated.	Calluses result in increased pressure on the foot. An ulcer may develop.
Myth #2	My foot problems are not serious because they are painless.	Patients with diabetes may have numbness in the feet. They do not feel pain, even when problems develop.
Myth #3	It is alright to test the temperature of water using my feet.	Diabetic patients may have numbness in their feet and will not be able to detect water at high temperatures. The feet may instead develop burns.
Myth #4	Diabetic wounds heal faster than normal.	Diabetic wounds typically heal slower than normal.

DID YOU REMEMBER TO...

❖ Check your feet daily for cuts, blisters, colour changes, swelling and in-grown toenails.
❖ Use a mirror to see soles of feet.
❖ Always wash feet with soap and water.
❖ Remember to wash between toes.
❖ Dry feet carefully using a soft towel.
❖ Use moisturizer to keep skin hydrated.
❖ Cut toenails straight across.
❖ Go for foot examination once a year.

AVOID

❖ Using hot water to wash your feet.
❖ Using a hot water bottle to warm your feet.
❖ Cutting calluses by yourself.
❖ Cutting nails too short.
❖ Leaving nails too long.
❖ Cutting out the corners of the nail.
❖ Digging down the sides of the nail bed.
❖ Walking around bare-foot.
❖ Wearing slippers all day.

Foot care when travelling

1. Flying to your destination

- Constantly sip water to avoid dehydration.
- Wear shoes with adjustable fittings.
- Ask for an aisle seat - walk up and down the aisle every half an hour to prevent your feet from swelling.
- Choose a seat with more legroom.

2. Upon Arrival

- Be careful of trolleys that might ramp onto feet.
- Arrange for a wheelchair if possible.
- Use a trolley - do not carry heavy luggage.

3. In subtropical or tropical countries

- Use insect repellant to avoid insect bites.
- Avoid eating, handling or exposing open wounds to raw seafood in areas where vibrio vulnificus is endemic (Bacteria which causes serious damage to the skin).
- Beware of rats which may nibble at your shoes and feet.
- Do not go barefoot when walking on the beach or in the sea.
- Use sun block with high SPF to protect your skin.
- Keep dry skin moisturised.

6

3. A Patient's Guide to Footwear

Aziz Nather and Zest Ang Yi Yen

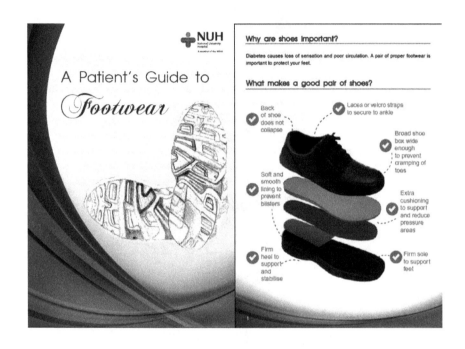

What type of shoe should you avoid wearing?

❖ Slip-on shoes

• Excessive movement causes friction.

❖ Slippers

• No protection over toes and heels.
• Increases friction between toes.

❖ High-heeled shoes

• No back support.
• Too much pressure on forefoot.

❖ Shoes with tight shoe boxes

• Cause cramping of toes.

❖ Thin-soled shoes

• Lack adequate protection and shock absorption.

Do's and Don'ts when selecting a pair of shoes

Do's	Don'ts
Shop later in the day	Don't buy shoes that perfectly fit your foot

Your feet swell throughout the day. Shop in the afternoon or night when your feet are at their maximum size.

Don't buy shoes that does not have enough toe space.

Try shoes with socks	Don't buy shoes made of synthetic materials

Socks add one more layer of padding. Wearing socks ensures that your shoe fits properly.

Avoid materials like PVC, polyurethane or rubber. Purchase leather or suede shoes.

Do's	Don'ts
Buy shoes that fit the larger foot	Don't wear new shoes for a long time to break in

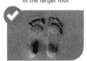

Your left and right feet are of different sizes. Buy shoes fitting the larger foot.

Break into your shoes slowly. Start by wearing your shoes for 30 min each day. Check for blisters, cuts or calluses each time.

Choose shoes without interior seams	Don't select a shoe based on pre-measured shoe sizes

Interior seams may rub against your foot and cause blisters.

Try each pair of new shoes carefully to ensure a proper fit.

Before wearing your shoes

1. Wear cotton socks

❖ To absorb moisture and prevent friction. Cotton allows your feet to breathe.
❖ Change your socks regularly.
❖ Do not wear knee-high socks or socks with elastic tops.

2. Check shoes for wear and tear

❖ Check both the inside and outside of your shoes.
❖ Replace your shoes when they are worn out.

3. Check the inside and outside of your shoes for foreign bodies or for damage to shoes

❖ Shake pebbles and grit from shoes before putting them on.
❖ Replace your shoes if they are worn out.

Common Myths

Myth 1: It is alright to go barefoot at home.

- ❖ Wear soft cushioned slippers at home to protect your feet.
- ❖ Wear covered shoes when outdoors.

Myth 2: Massage slippers improve blood circulation.

- ❖ They increase pressure over sole of foot and can cause your skin to breakdown.

Myth 3: We only need one pair of shoes.

Alternate between two pairs of shoes regularly.

- ❖ This allows each pair to air completely.
- ❖ This prevents each pair from wearing out quickly.

Myth 4: Shoes should fit snugly around entire foot.

- ❖ Leave one thumb's space between longest toe and the front of the shoe.

6

Section 8

Supplement for Nurses & Podiatrists

Chapter 21

Team Approach for Diabetic Foot

Aziz Nather

Introduction

The guidelines and recommendations entitled "Diabetes and Foot Care: Time to Act" published by the International Diabetes Federation and International Working Group on Diabetic Foot showed that a 60% reduction in amputation rate could be achieved through a combination of a multidisciplinary team approach and education in foot care and footwear.[1] Faglia E. *et al.*[2] showed that the formation of a "Foot Team" running "Foot Clinic" reduced major amputation rate from 40% to 23.5% (1998). A study by Driver V. R. *et al.*[3] also indicated that the formation of a "Specialised Foot Care Clinic" decreased the amputation rate dramatically from 9.9 per 1,000 to 1.8 per 1,000 over 5 years (2005).

A Multidisciplinary Team

Members

For optimal management of diabetic foot problems, a Multidisciplinary Diabetic Foot Team (Figure 1)[4] would comprise the following:

- ✓ Orthopaedic surgeon
- ✓ Endocrinologist
- ✓ Infectious disease specialist

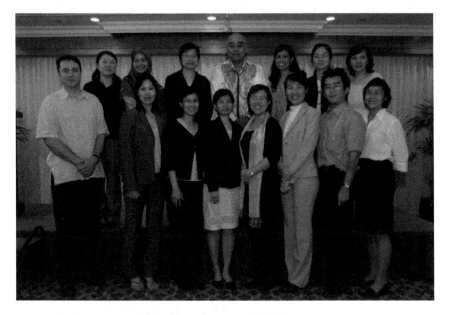

Figure 1:   Pioneers of NUH Team

- ✓ Podiatrist
- ✓ Wound care nurse
- ✓ Diabetic care nurse
- ✓ Case manager
  - Manages the clinical pathway for diabetic foot problems — this is strategic to the success of the team
- ✓ Dietitian, occupational therapist, physical therapist, and medical social worker

The patient care process involving various members of the team is shown in Figure 2.

Function of a Multidisciplinary Team

Weekly Team Round

In NUH, a Weekly Team Ward Round is carried out to ensure the patients have optimal glycaemic control, appropriate antibiotic coverage,

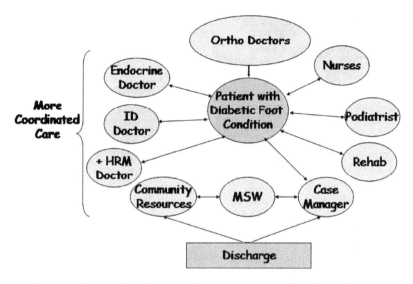

Figure 2:   Patient Care Process with Implementation of a Clinical Pathway

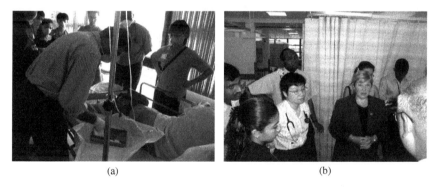

(a)   (b)

Figure 3:   (a) Weekly Grand Ward Rounds at NUH; (b) Ward Round with Visiting Consultant, Ali Foster, King's College, London, in October 2003

follow-up on any surgical intervention performed, podiatric care, education on diabetes, foot care and footwear, and an appropriate discharge plan. Such rounds allow for total patient care with input from all relevant specialists in the team to arrive at a complete plan for the day-to-day management of the patient[4] (Figure 3).

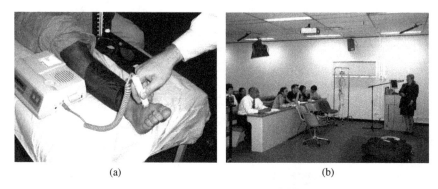

(a)   (b)

Figure 4:   (a) Teaching Session at NUH Showing ABI Measurement; (b) Guest Lecture by Ali Foster, October 2003, During NUH Foot Team Teaching Session

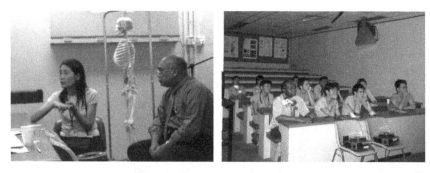

Figure 5:   Briefing on Clinical Pathway to House Officers and Medical Officers in NUH

Multidisciplinary Teaching Sessions

The NUH team conducted multidisciplinary teaching sessions (Figure 4) each month. Topics covered all relevant disciplines, including endocrine control, microbiological aspects, orthopaedic aspects, wound care, podiatric care, foot screening, and the role of vascular surgery.

Clinical Pathway

In addition to the formation of a team of specialists, Martinez D.A. *et al.*[5] showed that the implementation of a Clinical Pathway was instrumental to the high quality of services provided in a general hospital (2004).

In NUH, the case manager in the team implemented and monitored the pathway, ensuring that full compliance was obtained from all house officers and medical officers in all wards (Figures 5 and 6). The pathway

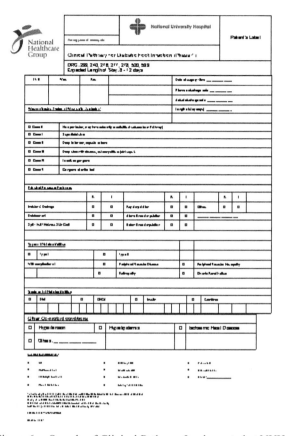

Figure 6:   Sample of Clinical Pathway Implemented at NUH

was started in the emergency department or in wards where patients were admitted. Upon admission, the DFP is classified according to King's classification[6] (Stage 1: Normal Foot; Stage 2: High-risk Foot; Stage 3: Ulcerated Foot; Stage 4: Cellulitic Foot; Stage 5: Necrotic Foot; Stage 6: Major Amputation). The house officer would also be required to do baseline investigations and to initiate the necessary referrals to the podiatrist and other members of the diabetic foot team where necessary.

Surgery

In our team, the need for surgery is discussed with the whole team after input from vascular surgeons, orthopaedic surgeons, infectious disease specialists, podiatrists, and nurses.

Outpatient Clinics

A weekly diabetic foot clinic is conducted by an orthopaedic surgeon together with a podiatrist and diabetic wound care nurse to provide further care for and follow-up for patients discharged.

Patient Education

In NUH, the team round is the starting point for nurses and podiatrists to provide all patients with individualised education sessions on diabetes care, foot care, and footwear. Patient education pamphlets on care of diabetes, care of foot, and choice of footwear developed by the team are given to all patients.

Outcome of a Multidisciplinary Team Approach (Figure 2)

Amputation Rates

Major amputation rate in NUH was significantly reduced from 31.15% to 11.01% from 2002 to 2007 after a multidisciplinary diabetic foot team was combined with a clinical pathway.[4]

Complication Rates

In the case of NUH, a significantly lower complication rate in 2005, 2006, and 2007 (after team formation) of about 6.1%–7.3% was found as compared to 19.7% in 2002 (before team formation).[4]

Costs

The NUH team found a reduction in mean hospitalisation cost per patient (though not statistically significant) from $8,847.17 in 2002 (pre-team formation) to $8,383.79 in 2007 (post-team formation).[4]

However, a fall in amputation rate reduces related cost in terms of loss of productivity, disability, and premature mortality. This will therefore contribute to reducing the total economic cost.

References

1. K. Bakker, A. Foster, W. Van Houtum, and P. Riley, *Diabetics and Foot Care: Time to Act*, International Diabetes Federation, Belgium, p. 34 (2005).
2. E. Faglia, F. Favales, A. Aldeghi, P. Calia, A. Quarantiello, P. Barbano, M. Puttini, B. Palmieri, G. Brambilla, A. Rampoldi, E. Mazzola, L.Valenti, G. Fattori, V. Rega, A. Cristalli, G. Oriani, M. Michael, and A. Morabito, Change in major amputation rate in a center dedicated to diabetic foot care during the 1980s: prognostic determinants for major amputation, *J Diabetes Complications.* **12**(2): 96–102 (1998).
3. V. R. Driver, J. Madsen, and R. A. Goodman, Reducing amputation rates in patients with diabetes at a military medical center: The limb preservation service model. *Diabetes Care.* **28**(2): 248–253 (2005).
4. A. Nather, S.B. Chionh, K.L. Wong, X.B.V. Chan, L. Shen, P.A. Tambyah, A. Jorgensen, and A. Nambiar, Value of team approach combined with clinical pathway for diabetic foot problems: a clinical evaluation, *Diabet Foot Ankle.* **1**: 5731–5740 (2010).
5. D.A. Martinez, J.I. Aquayo, G. Morales, M.I. Aguirán, and F. Illán, Impact of a clinical pathway for the diabetic foot in a general hospital [Spanish]. *Ann Med Int.* **21**(9): 420–424 (2004).
6. M.E. Edmonds and A.V.M. Foster, *Managing the Diabetic Foot*, 2nd Edition, Blackwell Science, Oxford (2005).

Chapter 22

Managing Diabetic Foot Ulcers — A Nursing Perspective

Gulnaz Tariq

Introduction

Diabetes is one of the fast-growing non-communicable disease. Diabetes can lead to many complications, such as foot ulcers and amputations.

Control of diabetes is needed to avoid complications. It is important to know the risk factors of developing foot ulcers to avoid it to happen.

Prevention strategies are the key factor to prevent the development of foot ulcers.[1-3]

Education to patient with diabetes is required to have success in prevention strategies.

Identification of the At-Risk Foot

History

Taking history is the baseline factor for identifying the at-risk foot.[1-3] Following are the important elements that clinicians should ask:

- History of previous foot ulceration or deformity, thickening of the skin or callous, blistering, and bleeding.
- It is important to know if the person can perform foot hygiene by self or with assistance of others.

- Type of shoe that person is wearing and frequency of usage.
- To ask if they are wearing eyeglasses or having poor vision as this will be barrier to do self-inspection and may not be aware of the foot condition and problems.
- To know if they feel some tingling sensation, numbness, or loss of sensation on the feet. Person may not be aware of feeling that the shoes is not fitting well and there are some problems developed on the feet.

Holistic Assessment

The holistic assessment of patients with diabetes and foot ulceration should include the following:[1,2]

- History of present illness
  - o How the ulcer or injury happened? (from trauma or shoes, etc.)
  - o Period of ulceration
  - o Treatments provided
  - o Results of the treatments
- Past medical history
- Medications
- Present diabetes management
- Allergies
- Family history of diabetes
- Activities of daily living
- Quality of life

Skin Conditions

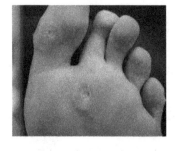 Skin is one of the affected parts of the body when you are having diabetes. Fortunately, most of the skin conditions can be prevented or easily treated if found out early.

Skin callus is the most common skin that you will see on person with diabetes. This is a thickened skin that occurs due to response to stress, pressure, friction, or sheering forces from ill-fitting footwear.

Dark red streaks especially in the centre of calluses are considered a pre-ulcerative lesion.

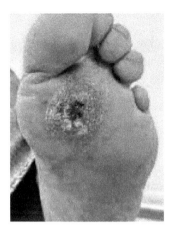

There are some skin conditions that you can notice that include the following:

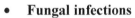

- **Bacterial infections**
  Bacteria can enter the body through an opening in your skin, such as wounds or ulcers.

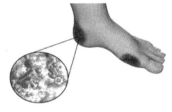

- **Fungal infections**
  There are two common superficial fungal infections in person with diabetes.
  1. **Tinea pedis or athlete's foot**
     Fungal infection that usually begins between the toes.
  2. **Onychomycosis**
     Fungal infection of the nails that causes discolouration, thickening, and separation from the nail bed.

1. Tinea pedis or athlete's foot

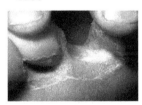

2. Onychomycosis

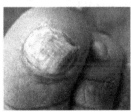

- **Itching**
  Itching of the feet is common in people
  with diabetes as a result of high sugar
  levels over a long period of time.

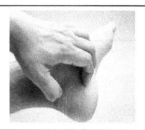

Other skin problems happen mostly or only to people with diabetes. These include the following:

- **Diabetic dermopathy**
  It is known for small lesions or spots on the
  skin. Person with diabetes can have this skin
  condition that can appear anywhere on the
  body but tends to develop on bony parts, such
  as the shins.

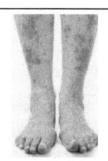

- **Necrobiosis lipoidica diabeticorum**
  Rash that occurs in the lower legs.

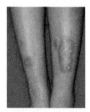

- **Diabetic blisters**
  Person with diabetes might experience blisters
  on their skin. These are relatively rare but
  reports on how often they develop differ.
  Blisters typically occur in people who do not
  control blood sugar well.

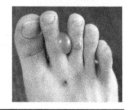

Nursing Consideration for Skin Conditions

Assessing the skin of a person with diabetes will give an early indication of the circulatory and neurological status as well as ulceration risk. They

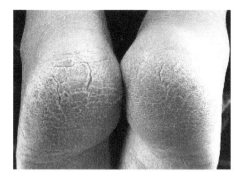

Figure 1:   Dry Skin Over Back of Both Heels with Fissuring.

are more prone to ulceration and infection than non-diabetics. Routine skin assessment allows the detection of early changes.[2]

Hygiene

Poor hygiene of the foot can occur when a person is unable to physically care for their feet. Skin that is too dry can lead to fissures (Figure 1) whereas skin that is too moist can results in fungal infection in between the toes. Any disruption on the skin integrity can be a portal of entry for infection.

Nursing Consideration for Hygiene

Make sure that feet should be clean and free from any dirt. Skin of a person with diabetes should maintain intact and avoid possible injury related to friction forces associated with wearing shoes and ambulation. Application of fragrance-free lotion or cream can help maintain dry skin supple. Maintaining appropriate care and cut of toenails is an important aspect of personal hygiene. Person with thick and hard nails may require assistance with nail care.[2]

Deformity

Inspection and assessment of the feet are necessary to observe for conditions for which the person with diabetes may or may not be aware.

There are several foot deformities that resulted from diabetes such as the following:

- **Charcot foot**
  One of the serious complications of diabetes that caused bone destruction.

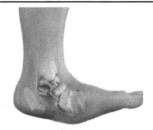

- **Hallux valgus**
  It is a lateral deviation of the first toe and may be accompanied by overlapping toes.

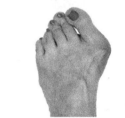

- **Toe deformities**
  - **Claw toes**
    Toes bent into an abnormal claw-like shape.
  - **Hammer toes**
    It is the presence of abnormal bend in its middle joint, making the toe bend downward to look like a hammer.
  - **Mallet toes**
    It refers to an upward bend at the toe joint.

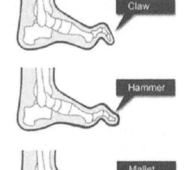

Nursing Consideration for Deformity

These deformities may benefit from appropriate footwear or padding to prevent skin breakdown and ulceration. Referral to orthopedics will be helpful to correct the deformity through surgery.[2]

Footwear and Device

Check and look at the existing footwear and devices that a person with diabetes uses. It should examine for areas of pressure and adherence when wearing. Comprehensive education should be given.[2]

- **Shoes:** Common cause of diabetic foot ulcers is caused by improper footwear. Tight shoes over the bones of the foot will increase the chance of skin trauma. Following are the footwear tips when buying shoes.
  - Look for shoes that don't have pointed toes. Instead, choose "toe box" shoes to lessen the chance of corns, calluses, and blisters that can turn into ulcers.
  - Avoid high-heeled shoes because they put pressure on the ball of your foot and will cause balance issues which is not good if you have nerve damage.
  - Use shoes with lace rather than slip-ons. They provide better support and fit.
  - Buy the shoes at the end of the day because your feet are more likely to be a little swollen. Choose at least half centimetre bigger size shoe.
- **Keep your shoes on:** Make sure that when you find the shoes that fit you well, suggest to wear them all the time. Don't go barefoot to avoid injury or ulcerations.
- **Orthotics:** Orthotics are custom-made inserts to apply to the shoe. It will help relieve the pressure on the foot.

Nursing Consideration for Footwear and Device

Wearing appropriate shoes can help reduce risk and promote healthy circulation in your feet.[2]

Qualities of a Good Dressing Protocol

- Select a correct dressing or therapy based on product description, evidence, availability, funding, available resources, clinician education, and patient acceptance.[2]

- Develop a customised management protocol based on the location and availability of resources and services.
- Communicate the plan, including the length of time of product use, regular reports, images, and photos as needed.
- Communicate to clinicians, caregivers, and patients the management protocol and provide follow-up information, including written and/or verbal communication to the team.
- Initiate the management protocol, ensuring there are built-in standardised assessment parameters to measure progress towards the identified goals of care.
- Evaluate the impact of the management protocol to identify met and unmet goals of care.
- Reassess the management plan at least every 2–4 weeks and more often if required to avoid long-term use of dressing/therapies with no evidence of improvement.

Patient Education on Foot Care

Diabetic foot care is important to prevent injury and ulceration. Diabetes may cause nerve damage that takes away the feeling in your feet. Due to these problems, you may not notice a foreign object in your shoe. To avoid serious foot complications, follow the following recommendations:[2]

o **Inspect your feet daily:** Check your feet for any possible injuries such as cuts, blisters, redness, and swelling or nail problems. You can use a hand mirror to look at the bottom of your feet. Make sure to inform your doctor if you notice anything.
o **Wash your feet with lukewarm water. Never use hot water:** Washing your feet daily will keep them clean. Check first the temperature of water before using it to clean your feet.
o **Clean your feet with care and be gentle:** Clean your feet using a soft washcloth or sponge. Avoid strong rubbing to prevent friction that will cause skin injury. Pat to dry the feet and dry them in between the toes carefully.
o **Moisturise your feet but not between your toes:** Application of fragrance-free moisturiser will keep your skin healthy. Daily moisturising will keep dry skin from itching or cracking. But don't

moisturise in between the toes to avoid development of fungal infection.

o **Cut nails carefully:** Cut them straight across and file the edges. Don't cut nails too short, as this could lead to ingrown toenails. If you have concerns about your nails, consult your doctor.

o **Never treat corns or calluses yourself:** Visit your doctor or podiatrist for appropriate treatment.

o **Wear clean and dry socks:** Make sure to change them daily.

o **Choose socks that are made specifically for person with diabetes:** These special socks have extra cushioning and do not have elastic tops. They are higher than the ankle and are made from fibres that makes the moisture away from the skin.

o **Wear socks to bed:** If your feet get cold at night, wear socks. Never use a heating pad or a hot water bottle to avoid skin jury or even burn.

o **Inspect your shoes and feel the inside before wearing:** Remember that person with diabetes might not be able to feel pebbles or other foreign objects. Therefore, always inspect your shoes before putting them on to avoid injury.

o **Consider using an antiperspirant on the soles of your feet:** This is helpful if you have excessive sweating of the feet. If the antiperspirant is not helping, you can visit your dermatologist to treat excessive sweating of the feet.

o **Never walk barefoot:** Not even at home! Always wear shoes or appropriate slippers. You could step on something and get an injury or cut.

o **Take care of your diabetes:** Keep your blood sugar levels under control.

o **Do not smoke:** Smoking restricts blood flow in your feet.

o **Get periodic foot exams:** Seeing your foot and ankle doctor or podiatrist on a regular basis can help prevent foot complications of diabetes.

Conclusion

Diabetic foot ulcers can have serious complications, such as infection, amputation, and even death. Clinicians all over the world developed several prevention strategies to avoid complications. It is important to recognise early detection of skin changes or ulcer developments. Holistic assessment is vital in managing diabetic foot ulcers. Treat the patient as a whole and not only the hole in the patient. However, multidisciplinary team is an essential factor to provide appropriate management. Person with diabetes should understand the disease and agree with the treatment plan. Patient education is important.

References

1. M. Botros *et al.*, Best practice recommendations for the prevention and management of diabetic foot ulcers, *Foundations of Best Practice for Skin and Wound Management*, Wounds Canada (2021).
2. Registered Nurses' Association of Ontario (RNAO), *Clinical Best Practice Guidelines: Assessment and Management of Foot Ulcers for People with Diabetes*, 2nd Edition (2013).
3. J.L. Kuhnke, M. Botros, J. Elliot, E. Rodd-Nielsen, H. Orsted, and R.G. Sibbald, The case for diabetic foot screening, *Wound Care Canada*. **1**(2): 1–7 (2013).

Chapter 23

Nutrition and Diabetes

Geoff Sussman

Nutrition plays a vital role in health and well-being for all people but especially for the diabetic or prediabetic. The major issues are good balanced nutrition for all diabetic patients with or without wounds, the importance of nutrition in gestational diabetes, and the impact of nutrition in wound healing.

There is a body of evidence to support the importance of diet to a diagnosed diabetic both Type 1 and Type 2. Evert *et al.* published recommendations for the management of adults with diabetes with the following goals[1]:

Goals of Nutrition Therapy that Apply to Adults with Diabetes[1]:
- To promote and support healthful eating patterns, emphasising a variety of nutrient-dense foods in appropriate portion sizes, in order to improve overall health and specifically to
  o attain individualised glycaemic, blood pressure, and lipid goals.

General recommended goals from the ADA for these markers are as follows:

- HbA1c — 7%.
- Blood pressure — 140/80 mmHg.

- LDL cholesterol — 100 mg/dL; triglycerides — 150 mg/dL; HDL cholesterol — 40 mg/dL for men; HDL cholesterol — 50 mg/dL for women.
- Achieve and maintain body weight goals.
- Delay or prevent complications of diabetes.

In relation to people with prediabetes, a consensus report by Evert *et al.* published recommendation goals as follows:[2]

Goals of Nutrition Therapy[2]:
- To promote and support healthful eating patterns, emphasising a variety of nutrient-dense foods in appropriate portion sizes, to improve overall health and specifically to
  - improve HbA1c, blood pressure, and cholesterol levels (goals differ for individuals based on age, duration of diabetes, health history, and other present health conditions).
- Further recommendations for individualisation of goals can be found in the ADA Standards of Medical Care in Diabetes[3]:
  - Achieve and maintain body weight goals.
  - Delay or prevent complications of diabetes.
- To address individual nutrition needs based on personal and cultural preferences, health literacy and numeracy, access to healthful food choices, willingness, and ability to make behavioural changes, as well as barriers to change.
- To maintain the pleasure of eating by providing positive messages about food choices, while limiting food choices only when indicated by scientific evidence.
- To provide the individual with diabetes with practical tools for day-to-day meal planning.

The prevalence of gestational diabetes is rising[4] and these patients need to be advised on their diet not only during the pregnancy but also as an ongoing issue to minimise the risk of developing diabetes years later.

Nutrition plays an essential role in wound healing and wound care practices, and nutritional support needs to be considered a fundamental part of wound management. Attending to nutrition in wound care is also cost-effective.

Poor nutrition before or during the healing process may delay healing and impair wound strength, making the wound more prone to breakdown.

Neglecting the nutritional health of an individual with a wound can compromise the entire wound management process. Chronic wounds may occur in any individual but are more frequent in the elderly and chronically ill. With an ageing population and a dramatically increasing prevalence of chronic disease, wound care will inevitably become an even more significant issue for health systems.

A wound causes several changes in the body that can affect the healing process, including changes in energy, protein, carbohydrate, fat, vitamin, and mineral metabolism. When the body sustains a wound, stress hormones are released in a fight-or-flight reaction and the metabolism alters to supply the injured area with the nutrients it needs to heal — known as the catabolic phase.

The body experiences an increased metabolic rate, loss of total body water, and increased collagen and cellular turnover. These effects can be pronounced even with a small wound.

The Role of Nutrition and Wound Healing

- The role of nutrition in wound healing has been known for hundreds of years. Poor nutritional intake and the lack of essential nutrients significantly alter the body's ability to heal wounds.
- Adequate nutrition is essential in individuals with diabetic foot ulceration (DFU); therefore, an assessment of dietary intake is critical. A lack of nutrients including protein, zinc, and vitamins C and D has all been associated with poor wound healing. However, the comprehensive dietary intake of Australian adults with DFU is poorly understood.[5,6]

  Calories refer to the total number of calories, or "energy", supplied from all sources (carbohydrate, fat, protein, and alcohol) in one serving of the food. To achieve or maintain a healthy body weight, you should balance the number of calories you consume with the number of calories your body uses and balance higher-calorie meals with ones with fewer calories.
- Protein and DNA synthesis are essential elements of the healing process. Any diminution of the building blocks (i.e. amino acids and nucleic acids) or any cofactors involved in these processes can have detrimental effects on the wound.
- Malnutrition of any sort can have a negative effect, but protein deficiency has a significant impact on healing, due to the importance

of collagen synthesis during healing. Low protein results in decreased fibroblast proliferation, decreased proteoglycan and collagen synthesis, decreased angiogenesis, and altered collagen remodelling.[5]

- Albumins are very important and if a level of less than 1.5 mg/dL, this will result in poor collagen production and overall poor wound healing.
- Malnutrition can exist well before and after wounding.
- Vitamin deficiencies can also lead to poor healing, especially vitamins C and D. Vitamin C is essential in collagen formation, and deficiencies lead to decreased crosslinking and reduced tissue tensile strength.[5,6]

Macronutrients

- Fluids
- Fat
- Carbohydrates
- Protein

Fluids

Chronic wounds can be very exudative, and the loss of fluid daily can amount to litres. The replacement of such fluid and often albumin and electrolytes is not usually considered part of the management of the wound. Severe systemic oedema continues to be a major complication following burn injury. Although attempts have been made to limit oedema formation by modifying the resuscitative regimen, no single fluid resuscitation formula has proven to be superior.[6,7]

Staying well hydrated, mainly through drinking ample amounts of plain water (6–8 glasses a day for most adults) also helps our immune system. Drinking plain water instead of sugar-sweetened beverages also helps reduce the risk of consuming too many calories for maintaining a healthy weight. In patients with highly exudating wounds, a fluid balance chart should be considered.

Fat

Fats, including mono- and polyunsaturated fats, provide fuel for wound healing. Fats are a safe and concentrated source of energy. For example, fat has more energy at 9 cal/g than carbohydrate at 5 cal/g. Importantly, adequate fats are needed to prevent the body from using protein for energy.

Fatty acids are a major component of cell membranes and demands for essential fatty acids increase after injury.

Essential unsaturated fatty acids must be supplied in the diet as the body cannot synthesise enough for the needs of wounds. The benefit of omega-3 fatty acid supplementation in wound healing is still not clear and there is some evidence this may reduce wound strength.

High fat intake can result in fatty infiltration of the liver. An excess of omega-3 fatty acids may turn into immunosuppression; this can be a complicating factor in wound patients who have local or systemic infection. Also, an excess of omega-6 fatty acids may exacerbate. Protein is essential for the maintenance and repair of body tissue. Depleted protein levels will cause inflammation which needs to be controlled.[6,7]

Carbohydrates

Carbohydrate is a major source of calories for use by the body, and its availability is essential to prevent other nutrients (e.g. protein) from being converted into energy. But increased carbohydrate intake provides energy that is essential for optimal healing. This needs to be undertaken with caution in people with diabetes, and monitoring (e.g. blood glucose levels and glycated haemoglobin) will be required.[6–8]

Protein

Protein is essential for the maintenance and repair of body tissue. Depleted protein levels will cause a decrease in collagen development, slowing the wound-healing process. Adequate protein levels will help achieve optimal wound healing rates. Protein requirements should be calculated on an individual basis, and they should be monitored closely.

This needs to happen along with the provision of calories because if energy needs aren't met, the body will use protein for energy rather than for wound healing.

This needs to happen along with the provision of calories because if energy needs aren't met, the body will use protein for energy rather than for wound healing. In slow-to-heal/chronic wounds, a recommended daily intake of 1.5 g/kg/day will meet the protein needs of most individuals but up to 3 g/kg/day may be appropriate for those with more severe wounds.[6–8]

Sources of protein include red and white meats, fish, eggs, liver, dairy products (milk, cheese, and yoghurt), soybeans, legumes, seeds, nuts, and grains.

L-arginine is an amino acid that has several properties that enhances several pathways involved in wound healing, such as its role in structural protein synthesis.[9]

As the body needs more protein during wound healing, the demand for normally non-essential amino acids, such as L-arginine, becomes essential.

Dietary supplementation with arginine has been shown to enhance protein metabolism, helping decrease muscle loss and collagen synthesis, which helps increase the strength of the wound; in addition, L-arginine is essential for the stimulation of the nitric oxide pathway, which is in turn important for collagen deposition in wound healing.

L-arginine supplementation has also been shown to enhance the immune system and improve the secretion of growth hormone and insulin that are also involved in wound healing supplementing with 9 g of L-arginine has been shown to promote wound healing. An average dietary intake provides about 4 g L-arginine/day. Arginine is conditionally essential, meaning that when we are healthy, our bodies produce sufficient arginine; however, during healing, requirements increase to a level where supplementation is recommended.[9]

Excess protein may cause serious metabolic complications. These include acidosis. In surplus protein feeding, the nitrogen of the amino acids is broken down to ammonia and then urea. Increased renal urea excretion requires appropriate water excretion. Overfeeding protein with inadequate water can produce hypertonic dehydration.

Micronutrients

Micronutrients act as cofactors in many pathways and are critical to all activities of macronutrients. Included in micronutrients are the following:

- Vitamins
- Minerals
- Trace Elements

Vitamin A

Vitamin A increases the inflammatory response in wounds, stimulating collagen synthesis.

Low vitamin A levels can result in delayed wound healing and susceptibility to infection.

It has also been shown that vitamin A can restore wound healing impaired by long-term steroid therapy or by diabetes. Serious stress or injury can cause an increase in vitamin A requirements. While the mechanisms of vitamin A in wound healing are still not well understood, it plays an important role.

Supplementation with vitamin A requires caution, as there is a risk of toxicity.

Vitamin A is found in milk, cheese, eggs, fish, dark green vegetables, oranges, red fruits, and vegetables. The recommended dose in cases of vitamin A deficiency is 700–3000 IU — the higher range is for males.[6-8]

Vitamin C

Vitamin C plays an important role in collagen synthesis and subsequent crosslinking, as well as the formation of new blood vessels (angiogenesis). Adequate vitamin C levels help strengthen the healing wound.

Vitamin C also has important antioxidant properties that help the immune system, and it increases the absorption of iron.

Vitamin C deficiency impairs wound healing and has also been associated with an increased risk of wound infection. Research has shown vitamin C supplementation helps promote pressure ulcer healing. Recommended vitamin C supplementation for deficient patients is 60–200 mg daily. Doses over 200 mg a day are not necessary as tissue saturation occurs at this point.[6-8]

Vitamin D

For many years, it was known that vitamin D regulated the level of calcium in the body. In the last 10 years, research has shown that it plays a much larger role in the body in maintaining our health. In fact, it was found to have an extensive impact on the organs, tissues, and cells in the body.

Vitamin D in fact is not a vitamin, it is a hormone; it plays an increasingly important role in many aspects of the body's functions. A lack of this hormone has been shown to be a major factor in the development of multiple sclerosis and has a major influence in preventing cancers, influenza, autism, asthma, cardiovascular diseases, and diabetes.

The protective effects of vitamin D are mediated through the regulation of several components, such as the immune system and calcium homeostasis. However, an increasing amount of evidence suggests that vitamin D also affects ß cells directly thereby rendering them more resistant to the types of cellular stress encountered during T1D and T2D. This review evaluates the role of vitamin D signalling in the pathogenesis of T1D and T2D with a special emphasis on the direct effects of vitamin D on pancreatic ß cells. Insulin secretion is a process dependent on changes in intracellular calcium concentration. The effects of vitamin D on ß cells may be by its regulation of extracellular calcium and calcium flux through the ß cell, or through calcium-independent pathways. Whether or not acting independently, vitamin D or calcium deficiency may alter the balance between intracellular and extracellular calcium in ß cells, interfering with insulin secretion and possibly synthesis.[6–8,10,11]

Other Micronutrients

Micronutrients have a range of functions to prevent oxidative damage to polyunsaturated fatty acids in cell membranes and to DNA within all cells. Zinc, iron, and trace elements are all involved in the superoxide dismutase enzymes in mitochondria and the cytoplasm, and selenium is part of the glutathione peroxidase enzyme system, which helps dispose of hydrogen peroxide. Zinc is a trace element, present in small amounts in the body, which has a well-established role in wound healing.[6–8]

Zinc

Zinc plays a key role in protein and collagen synthesis, and in tissue growth and healing.

Zinc deficiency has been associated with delayed wound healing, reduced skin cell production, and reduced wound strength.

Zinc deficiency is related to impaired wound healing, but there is controversy over the value of zinc supplements in surgical wounds, the best evidence relating to healing of cutaneous leg ulcers.

Zinc stimulates epithelialisation more than wound contraction in experimental wounds. In support of this, results from clinical trials indicate the beneficial effects of topical zinc on human wounds healing predominantly by epithelialisation.

Zinc levels of less than 100 μg/100 mL have been associated with impaired wound healing, but supplementation in people who are not zinc deficient generally has no benefit.[12]

Iron

The role of iron in preventing anaemia is well understood. However, iron's role in forming haemoglobin also means that it has a key role in optimising tissue perfusion, which is important throughout the healing process. It can also assist in collagen synthesis and is sourced from liver, red meat, fortified cereals, pulses, and green vegetables.

Iron deficiency can lead to impaired collagen crosslinking and reduced wound strength.

Iron is necessary for optimising tissue perfusion by transporting oxygen to the tissues and is necessary for collagen synthesis. A deficiency may cause increased tissue ischemia, impaired collagen crosslinking, and decreased wound strength. Possible symptoms of iron deficiency include loss of energy (mild fatigue to exhaustion), pallor, sore tongue, digestive tract disturbances, appetite disorders, and brittle spoon-shaped nails.[13]

Trace Elements

In addition to iron, copper and zinc have the closest relationship to wound healing. Copper is a required cofactor for cytochrome oxidase and the cytosolic antioxidant superoxide dismutase. Lysyl oxidase is a key copper enzyme used in the development of connective tissue, where it catalyses the crosslinking of collagen and strengthens the collagen framework.[14]

Summary

Nutrition plays a vital role in wound healing; every patient with a chronic wound needs a nutrition assessment. It is often not obvious that a patient may be malnourished and if possible, a dietitian would be helpful. Holistic wound care must include both nutritional support and supplementation where necessary, according to an individual's needs. It is important for all patients, but diabetic patients need a regular nutritional assessment.

A nutrient-rich diet is fundamental, but sometimes it is not possible to achieve adequate levels of essential nutrients through normal consumption of food and liquids. In these cases, nutritional supplementation has been shown to promote wound healing. Minimum standard of nutritional care encompasses three steps.[15,16]

References

1. A.B. Evert *et al.*, Nutrition therapy recommendations for the management of adults with diabetes, *J Hum Nutr Diet.* **35**: 786–790 (2022).
2. A.B. Evert *et al.*, Nutrition therapy for adults with diabetes or prediabetes: a consensus report, *Diabetes Care.* **42**: 731–754 (2019).
3. N. Namazi *et al.*, Nutrition and diet therapy in diabetes mellitus: a roadmap based on available evidence, *J Diabetes Metab Disorders.* **20**: 1913–1918 (2021).
4. T.L. Hernandez *et al.*, Nutrition therapy within and beyond gestational diabetes, *Diabetes Res Clin Pract.* **145**: 39–50 (2018).
5. R. Collins *et al.*, Macronutrient and micronutrient intake of individuals with diabetic foot ulceration: a short report, *J Hum Nutr Diet.* **35**: 786–790 (2022).
6. J.K. Stechmiller, Understanding the role of nutrition and wound healing, *Nutr Clin Pract.* **25**(1): 61–68 (2010).
7. S. Guo and L.A. DiPietro, Factors affecting wound healing, *J Dent Res.* **89**(3): 219–229 (2010).
8. P.D. Dworatzek *et al.*, Nutrition therapy, *Can J Diabetes.* **37**: S45–S55 (2013).
9. M.B. Witte and A. Barbul, Arginine physiology and its implication for wound healing, *Wound Repair Regen.* **11**: 419–423 (2003).
10. R. Razzaghi, The effects of vitamin D supplementation on wound healing and metabolic status in patients with diabetic foot ulcer, *J Diabetes Complications.* **31**: 766–772 (2017).
11. G.A. Pittas *et al.*, The role of vitamin D and calcium in type 2. Systematic review and meta-analysis, *J Clin Endocrinol Metab* **92**: 2017–2029 (2007).
12. A.B.G. Lansdown, U. Mirastschijski, N. Stubbs, E. Scanlon, and M.S. Ågren, Zinc in wound healing, *Wound Repair Regen.* **15**(1): 2–16 (2007).
13. J.A.Wright, T. Richards, and S.K.S. Srai, The role of iron in the skin and cutaneous wound healing, *Front Pharmacol. Drug Metab Transp.* **5**: Article 156 (2014).
14. T. Tuvemo and M. Gebre-Medhin, The role of trace elements in juvenile diabetes mellitus, *Pedriatrician.* **12**(4): 213–219 (1983).

15. M.J. Franz, J.L. Boucher, and A.B. Evert, Evidence-based diabetes nutrition therapy recommendations are effective: the key is individualization, *Diabetes, Metab Syndr Obesity: Targets Therapy.* **7**: 65–72 (2014).
16. R. Basiri *et al.*, Nutritional supplementation concurrent with nutrition education accelerates the wound healing process in patients with diabetic foot ulcers. *Biomedicines.* **8**: 263 (2020).

Chapter 24

Dressings and Alternative Therapies

Harikrishna K. R. Nair

Introduction

Good wound management is an important part of treating diabetic foot problems. Careful assessment of the wound and proper wound bed preparation are required before selecting the appropriate wound dressings.

Wound Bed Preparation

Wound bed preparation helps healing to occur more effectively, by identifying and removing the barriers to wound healing.[1] This speeds up endogenous wound healing and increases the effectiveness of treatment measures.[2] Wound bed preparation involves debridement, management of bacterial burden, and exudate management.

The TIME acronym (Table 1) adapted from the International Wound Bed Advisory Board[3] describes a framework for approaching wound bed preparation and suggests various management options based on clinical assessment of the wound.

The periwound skin also has to be assessed and managed as the epidermal cells or keratinocytes enter the wound bed from the periphery and help in wound healing. The Harikrishna Periwound Skin Classification (Table 2) was used in 2015 and then published in 2018 in the *International Journal of Wound Care*. The validation study was later published in the *Journal of Wound Care Silk Road Supplement* in 2020.

Table 1:   TIME Concept

Clinical Observations	Proposed Pathophysiology	Wound Bed Preparation Clinical Actions	Effect of Wound Bed Preparation	Clinical Outcome
Tissue non-viable or deficient	Defective matrix and cell debris impair healing	Debridement (episodic or continuous): • Autolytic, sharp surgical, enzymatic, mechanical, or biological • Biological agents	Restoration of wound base and functional extracellular matrix proteins	Viable wound base
Infection or inflammation	High bacterial counts or prolonged inflammation Inflammatory cytokines Protease activity Growth factor activity	Remove infected foci Topical/systemic: • Antimicrobials • Anti-inflammatories • Protease inhibition	Low bacterial counts or controlled inflammation: Inflammatory cytokines Protease activity Growth factor activity	Bacterial balance and reduced inflammation
Moisture imbalance	Desiccation slows epithelial cell migration Excessive fluid causes maceration of wound margin	Apply moisture-balancing dressings Compression, negative pressure or other methods of removing fluid	Restored epithelial cell migration, desiccation avoided Oedema, excessive fluid controlled, maceration avoided	Moisture balance
Edge of wound — non-advancing or undermined	Non-migrating keratinocytes Non-responsive wound cells and abnormalities in extracellular matrix or abnormal protease activity	Re-assess cause or consider corrective therapies: • Debridement • Skin grafts • Biological agents • Adjunctive therapies	Migrating keratinocytes and responsive wound cells. Restoration of appropriate protease profile	Advancing epidermal margin

Table 2:   Harikrishna Periwound Skin Classification

Grade	Type	Description
0		Normal Skin
1		At Risk Skin
2	A	Desiccation
(Exudate Centred)		
	B	Maceration
	C	Allergy
3		Inflammed
4		Infection
5		Atypical

Medical Management

The management of diabetic foot infections involves not just treatment of the wound itself but also medical management of the underlying causes. This includes the following:

- Endocrine or glycaemic control
- Medical nutrition therapy

Endocrine Control

Endocrine control is important as uncontrolled high blood glucose levels can impair wound healing. Hyperglycemia can affect the cellular response to tissue injury and limit the function of immune cells required for wound healing.[4,5] Patients with diabetic foot ulcers often have poor glycemic control. Control of blood glucose levels may be disrupted by the infection, surgical trauma, and physical stress that patients undergo.

Medical Nutrition Therapy

Good nutrition is vital for wound healing, as the healing wound relies on an adequate supply of nutrients. In patients with insufficient nutritional intake, Protein Energy Malnutrition (PEM) may occur. PEM is defined as a deficiency of protein and energy intake to meet bodily demands, and impedes the healing process.[6] It is often seen in elderly patients with chronic wounds.[7] Each patient's nutrition should be individualised based on their body weight, current medical status, as well as other premorbid conditions, such as obesity, hyperlipidemia, and hypertension. A dietitian or nutritionist should be involved. In patients who are kept fasting, carbohydrates should be provided using a 5% dextrose drip or dextrose/saline infusion.

Dressing of Diabetic Foot Ulcers

The purpose of a dressing is to

- protect the wound from trauma and microbial contamination,
- reduce pain,
- maintain temperature and moisture of wound,
- absorb drainage and debride the wound,
- control and prevent haemorrhage (pressure dressing),
- provide psychological comfort.

An ideal dressing should have these characteristics:

- able to remove excess exudates,
- be waterproof,
- able to maintain moist wound-healing environment,
- trauma protection,
- allows gaseous exchange if appropriate,
- non-adherent,
- provide barrier to pathogens,
- safe and easy to use,
- provide thermal insulation.

Types of Wound Dressings

The various types of wound dressings used in treating diabetic foot infections have different characteristics that allow them to be better suited for different types of wounds. The following Table 3 describes the characteristics and recommended uses for the different types of wound dressings.

Table 3: Types of Wound Dressings

Category	Characteristics	Recommendation
Film	Sterile, thin, waterproof, breathable, self-adhesive polyurethane film	Suitable for flat/shallow low exudate wound
Tulle dressing	Non-adherent dressing	Epithelialised low-exudate wound
Hydrocolloid	Adhesive dressing made of natural or synthetic polymer e.g. gelatin and pectin Forms a gel on contact with exudate	Suitable for flat/shallow low- to medium-exudate wound
Hydrogel	Amorphous, water-based gels or sheets rehydrate dry necrotic tissue	Suitable for dry, necrotic wound
Alginate	Forms a soft flexible gel	Suitable for moderately exudative lesion
Hydrofibre	Retains fluid within the structure of the fibre forming a soft gel	Suitable for cavity, deep or superficial wound with slough or eschar and medium to heavy exudate e.g. leg ulcer or pressure ulcer
Polyurethane foam	Available with or without an adhesive border	Suitable for granulating or epithelialising wound with moderate to heavy exudate
Silver dressing	Silver nano-particle or ion impregnated in a non-woven material that releases silver ions slowly	Suitable for critically colonised or infected wound
Iodine dressing	Povidone iodine impregnated in a non-woven material that releases iodine slowly	Suitable for critically colonised or infected wound

Topical oxygen therapies such as topical continuous oxygen and topical haemoglobin sprays have gained acceptance currently. Photobiomodulation utilising lasers has also been used to manage wounds and pain control. Microcurrent therapy is another modality for managing pain and accelerating wound closure by reducing inflammation and increasing perfusion.

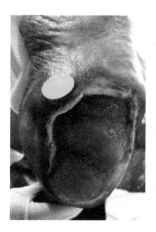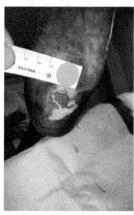

Figure 1.   Topical Haemoglobin Spray Applied (left) and a Wound Application was Used to Capture the Pictures and Analyse the Wound Healing Trajectory. Almost Complete Healing in Two Weeks.

How to Choose an Appropriate Dressing

The TIME framework for describing diabetic wounds can be used in the selection of wound dressings. Based on how well the tissue is healing and the amount of wound exudate, different dressing options can be used for the contact layer and outer layer. Different wound dressings may also be selected for different aims, such as treating the bacterial infection, maintaining adequate moisture balance, and promoting the advancement of the wound edge.

Table 4 describes how the TIME framework can be used in the selection of an appropriate dressing.

Adjunctive Therapies

In addition to dressing the wound appropriately, alternate forms of treatment may be used as adjuncts to aid in wound healing.

Table 4: TIME Framework in Selection of Appropriate Dressing

| | Aim of Care | Exudate | Dressing | |
			Contact Layer	Outer Dressing
Tissue necrotic	If vascular supply is good, debride eschar and promote moisture balance	Dry or low	Hydrogel	Hydrocolloid or foam
		Moderate	Hydrocolloid	Gauze or film
		Heavy	Alginate, foam or hydrofibre	Gauze or foam with pad
	If vascular supply is compromised, keep eschar dry	Dry	Tulle gauze, film	Film or gauze
Sloughy	Deslough, provide moisture balance	Low	Hydrocolloid, hydrogel	Gauze or film
		Moderate	Alginate	Hydrocolloid with pad or gauze
		Heavy	Foam, hydrofibre	Foam with pad or gauze
			Negative Pressure Wound Therapy (NPWT)	
Granulating	Provide moisture balance	Low	Non-adherence material	Film or gauze
		Moderate	Hydrocolloid, foam	Gauze or contact layer with pad
			NPWT	
Epithelialising	Provide moisture balance	Low	Non-adherent material	Film or gauze
		Moderate	Hydrocolloid or foam	Gauze
Infection	Get rid of infection (biofilm)	Low	Nanocrystalline or ionic silver containing material, Iodine cream	Hydrocolloid with pad or gauze
		Moderate	Silver containing, iodine containing material	Foam with pad or gauze

(Continued)

Table 4   (*Continued*)

	Aim of Care	Exudate	Dressing	
			Contact Layer	**Outer Dressing**
Moisture balance	Maintain moist environment	Low	Film, hydrogel	Gauze
		Moderate	Hydrocolloid, alginate	Contact layer with pad or foam
		Heavy	Foam, hydrofibre, NPWT	Contact layer with pad or gauze
Edge	Promote advance of wound edge	Low	Film, hydrogel	Gauze
		Moderate	Hydrocolloid, alginate, NPWT	Contact layer with pad or foam
		Heavy	Foam, hydrofibre, NPWT	Contact layer with pad or gauze

Table 5:   Adjunctive Therapies

Technology	Mechanism	Indication	Recommendation
NPWT	Application of negative pressure to a wound in a closed environment. Maintains moist environment and prevents desiccation Promotes formation of granulation tissue	Open wound with high exudate	Reduces frequency of dressing changes. Offers temporary wound closure. Cannot be used in infected wound. Necrotic tissue should be debrided first
Hyperbaric oxygen	Provides 100% oxygen to the wound tissue	For wound with inadequate perfusion	Vascular supply is inadequate
Maggot debridement therapy Common green bottle fly (*Lucilia cuprina*)	Digestion of slough by secreting enzymes that dissolve the necrotic tissue and the biofilm	For wound with slough and necrotic tissue	For patients too ill to undergo surgical debridement
Hydrosurgery top	Ultra-thin, high-velocity stream of saline to debride with fine precision	For wound with slough or necrotic tissue	Useful for wound bed preparation

Table 5 describes the various types of adjunctive therapies and explains how they may help improve healing of the diabetic foot wound.

References

1. R.G. Sibbald, D. Williamson, H.L. Orsted *et al.*, Preparing the wound bed-debridement, bacterial balance, and moisture balance, *Ostomy Wound Manage.* **46**: 14–22 (2000).
2. *Paris Advisory Board* (June 2002).
3. G.S. Schultz, R.G. Sibbald, V. Falanga *et al.*, Wound bed preparation: a systematic approach to wound management, *Wound Repair Regen.* **11**(2 suppl): 1–28 (2003).
4. A. Terranova, The effects of diabetes mellitus on wound healing, *Plast Surg Nurs.* **11**(1): 20–25 (1991).
5. C.S. Rosenberg, Wound healing in the patient with diabetes mellitus, *Nurs Clin North Am.* **25**(1): 247–261 (1990).
6. R.H. Demling, Nutrition, anabolism and the wound healing process: an overview, *Eplasty.* **9**: e9 (2009).
7. R.M. Demling and L. DeSanti, Protein energy malnutrition and the non-healing cutaneous wound, *Medscape Education*, Article 418377 (2003).

Chapter 25

Negative Pressure Wound Therapy

Aziz Nather

Negative pressure wound therapy, also known as Vacuum Assisted Closure (VAC) therapy, is commonly used in the management of surgical wounds.

Basic Science

VAC therapy accelerates wound healing in several ways:

- *It provides a semi-occlusive environment that keeps the wound moist and clean*
  The moisture in the wound prevents desiccation. It also promotes migration and development of epithelial tissue.
- *It physically stimulates granulation tissue formation*
  The direct mechanical stress applied on the wound creates a biochemical effect at the cellular level. Cell division, angiogenesis, and granulation tissue formation are promoted.
- *It reduces wound exudate and decreases wound oedema*
  VAC therapy removes wound exudate. It also reduces extracellular fluid and oedema. Excess fluid at the wound can inhibit the proliferation of keratinocytes, endothelial cells, and fibroblasts — cells essential for wound healing. Proteases and cytokines in the wound fluid can cause continued inflammation of the wound. VAC therapy removes these.

- *It improves blood flow*
  VAC therapy facilitates optimal blood flow in the wound. This improves the delivery of oxygen, nutrients, and inflammatory mediators to the wound. Tissue perfusion is enhanced.
- *It alleviates infection by facilitating the removal of bacteria*

Application of VAC Dressing

A sterile polyurethane foam (GranuFoam) dressing is trimmed to fit into the wound (Figure 1(a)–(c)). The foam has a pore size of 400–600 μm to promote the in-growth of granulation tissue. Adhesive tape is used to cover the foam and surrounding skin (Figure 2). A non-collapsible tube

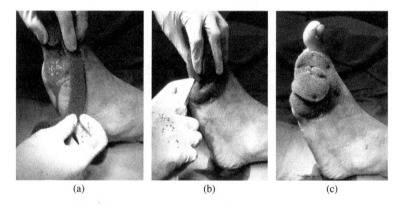

(a)   (b)   (c)

Figure 1:   (a)–(c) Step-by-Step Application of Foam to the Wound

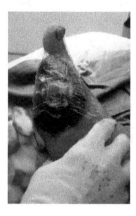

Figure 2:   Application of Adhesive Tape Over Foam and Surrounding Skin

connected to an electronic vacuum pump (Figure 3) is embedded in the foam (Figure 4).

Alternatively, a Bridge VAC dressing can be applied. In a Bridge VAC dressing, the GranuFoam dressing is placed over the wound and secured with adhesive drape. The bridge foam is then applied to allow placement of the suction pad away from the wound (Figure 5). By allowing placement of the suction pad outside the foot area, patients can wear protective shoes and walk with crutches.

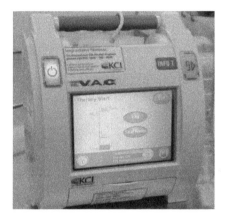

Figure 3: Electronic Vacuum Pump

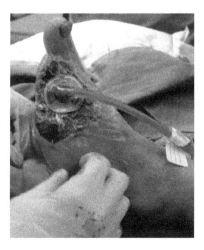

Figure 4: Completed VAC Dressing with the Non-collapsible Tube

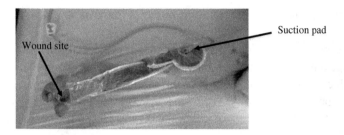

Figure 5:   Bridge VAC Dressing

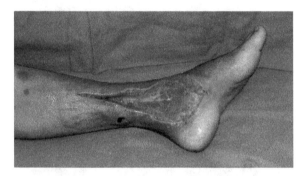

Figure 6:   Ankle Wound After Initial Surgical Debridement. The Medial Malleolus was Exposed in the Wound

After the application of either form of VAC dressing, negative pressure is then applied continuously or intermittently. At an optimal pressure of 125 mmHg, an alternating pressure cycle of 5 minutes turned on followed by 2 minutes turned off is carried out. Cyclical application of pressure is used to alter cell structures.

Case Study

A 60-year-old female developed necrotising fasciitis of the left ankle after minor trauma. Surgical debridement was performed. The large ulcer resulting from this aggressive wound debridement was treated with VAC therapy. Figures 6–8 show the progress of wound healing in the ulcer treated with VAC therapy. The ulcer eventually showed good healing. The healthy granulation bed allowed a split skin graft to be applied successfully (Figure 9).

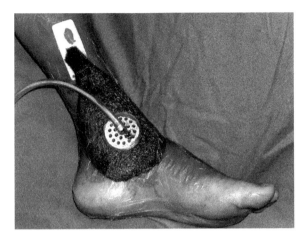

Figure 7:   VAC Therapy was Applied for 2 Weeks

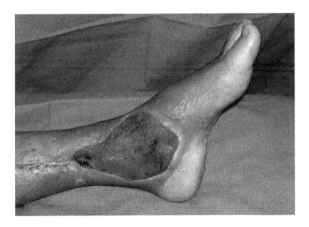

Figure 8:   Significant Healthy Stable Granulation Tissue Developed After 2 Weeks

In a study of 11 consecutive patients with diabetic foot problems treated by the NUH Diabetic Foot Team, the author found that VAC therapy facilitates healing in all cases.[1] The study was conducted from January 2008 to February 2009. The number of VAC dressings required ranged from 5 to 18 (one exceptional case required 37 dressings). The average length of treatment was 23.3 days. Nine wounds were closed with split skin grafting and two by secondary closure.

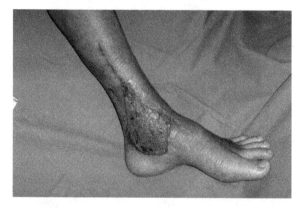

Figure 9:   Final Outcome After Split Skin Grafting at 1 Month Post Injury

Case Study 2

A 58-year-old Malay female presented with wet gangrene of the left second toe. ABI was 1.0 and TBI was 0.9. Both dorsalis pedis and posterior tibial pulses were palpable. A second ray amputation was performed. A Bridge VAC dressing was applied over the second ray amputation wound in the operating theatre. Bridge VAC dressing was used to allow this patient to put on footwear readily. From day 1 (Figure 10) to day 22 (Figure 11) of Bridge VAC dressing application:

- *Wound area* decreased by 12.5 cm² (41.7%)
  - o   Initial area (day 1): 30.0 cm²
  - o   Final area (day 22): 17.5 cm²
- *Granulation tissue* first appeared on day 4 till sufficient granulation was observed on day 22

A total of eight Bridge VAC dressings were used and a split skin graft was eventually performed after 22 days.

In a study of five consecutive cases of diabetic patients with foot ulcers, treated by the NUH Diabetic Foot Team, Bridge VAC dressing was found to be effective in all cases.[2] The study was conducted from May 2011 to October 2011. The number of dressings required ranged from 8 to 10. The average length of treatment was 33 days. Four wounds healed by split skin graft and one wound healed by secondary closure.

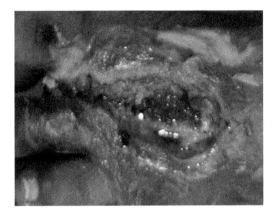

Figure 10:   Second Toe Ray Amputation Wound on Day 1

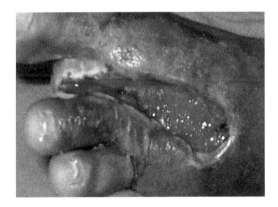

Figure 11:   Second Toe Ray Amputation Wound on Day 22

Innovative Techniques and NPWTi

White Foam

White foam dressings are far less porous and have been designed specially for use to fill tunnels and shallow undermining areas. It is also the foam dressing of choice for use in wounds with exposed bone, tendon, or surgical implants.

Veraflo Therapy (NPWTi)

Veraflo therapy uses dressings specially designed for instillation therapy — VAC Veraflo Cleanse Choice dressing.[3] This dressing is similar to VAC Granufoam dressing but is less hydrophobic and has greater strength to allow for better distribution of topical wound solutions across the wound bed.

Goals of therapy:
The goals using VAC Veraflo Cleanse Choice dressing[3] include the following:

- Cleansing wounds when areas of slough or non-viable tissue remain present on the wound surface
- Removing thick exudate
- Removing infectious materials
- Promoting granulation tissue formation

Therapy setting selection:
- Dwell time of 1 to 20 minutes.
- Negative pressure time phase of 30 minutes to 3.5 hours.
- Negative pressure of −125 or −150 mmHg.
- Topical solution volume will vary between wounds.
  Leow *et al.*[4] reported good results in the use of NPWTi using the waterfall technique in a case series in Sengkang General Hospital.

References

1. A. Nather, S.B. Chionh *et al.*, Effectiveness of vacuum-assisted closure (VAC therapy) in the healing of chronic diabetic foot ulcers, *Annals Acad Med Singapore*. **39**(5): 353–358 (2010).
2. A. Nather *et al.*, Effectiveness of Bridge VAC dressings in the treatment of diabetic foot ulcers, *Diabet Foot Ankle*. **2**: 5893–5901 (2011).
3. P.J. Kim *et al.*, Use of a novel foam dressing with negative pressure wound therapy and instillation: recommendations and clinical experience, *Wounds*. S1–S17 (2018).
4. K. Leow, J. Tey, A. Tan, K. Tan, and K.L. Wong, Negative pressure wound therapy with instillation and dwell time modifications for lower limb wounds with the waterfall technique: a case series, *Wounds: A Compend Clin Res Pract*. **32**(12): E12–E125 (2020).

Chapter 26

Maggot Debridement Therapy

Aziz Nather

Introduction

In the treatment of wounds by conventional wound dressings, alternative technologies could be used including negative pressure wound therapy, hyperbaric oxygen therapy, maggot debridement therapy, and hirudotherapy.

For debridement of wounds, alternative modalities include hydrosurgery debridement, ultra-sonic debridement, and maggot or leech therapy. Maggot therapy[1] is available in Singapore and Malaysia and could be used as an alternative to surgical debridement.

Basic Science

In maggot therapy, the larvae of *Lucilia cuprina* or *Lucilia sericata* are used to digest necrotic tissue, slough, and pathogens in the wound (Figure 1). About 3–10 sterile maggots are applied to each square centimetre of the wound surface. They are left within a cage-like dressing[2] or a biobag® dressing for 24–48 hours.

The cage-like dressing is made by first cutting a ring of hydrocolloid dressing, such as Duoderm (Figure 2). The hydrocolloid dressing is placed onto the skin surrounding the wound to protect the surrounding skin from maggot secretions. The maggots are added to the wound. A covering of porous dacron chiffon or a nylon stocking is then secured to the

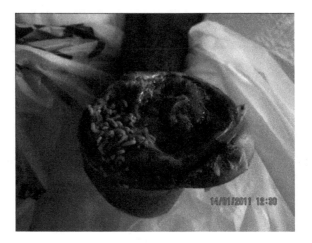

Figure 1:   Sterile Maggots Left on the Wound

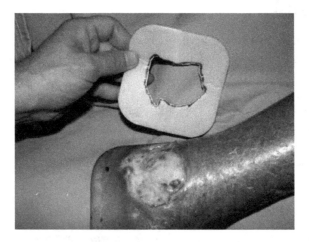

Figure 2:   A Cut Ring of Hydrocolloid Dressing is Placed Around the Wound

hydrocolloid ring with glue and tape. This cage-like dressing is then topped with a light gauze pad to absorb the necrotic drainage. The top layer of gauze is replaced every 4–6 hours.

Maggot therapy enhances wound healing in the following ways:

- *It provides wound debridement* — The maggot secretions and excretions contain powerful enzymes that lyse necrotic tissue without injuring healthy, viable tissues. One such degrading enzyme is trypsin. The maggots then ingest the lysed necrotic tissue.

- *It removes pathogens* — Maggot secretions contain antimicrobial substances that are bactericidal and capable of destroying biofilms.
- *It stimulates granulation tissue formation* — Maggot secretions contain substances, such as calcium carbonate, urea, allantoin, and ammonia. These substances promote granulation tissue formation and cellular migration. The mechanical stimulation of the wound surface by movements of maggots can also stimulate tissue growth.

Maggot therapy is especially useful for ulcers overlying joint capsules, bones, tendons, vessels, and nerves. These vital structures will not be debrided by the maggots.

Case Study 1

A patient had a wound following second, third, and fourth ray amputations. The wound extended over the dorsum and sole of the right foot (Figure 3).

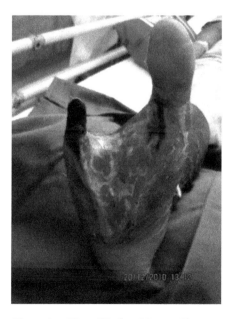

Figure 3:   Wound Before Maggot Therapy

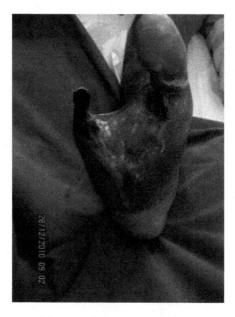

Figure 4:   Day 3 After First Application of Maggot Therapy

It was subjected to maggot therapy. Figure 4 shows the ability of maggot therapy to remove slough, leaving behind good granulation tissue.

Case Study 2

A 68-year-old Malay female with diabetes mellitus was admitted with cellulitis of the left foot. ABI was 1.2 and TBI was 0.7. Neuropathy was present with an abnormal VPT reading (32V) and monofilament test reading (7/10). The patient presented with erythema and a blister over the lateral aspect of the left foot. Wound cultures were positive for Pseudomonas *aeruginosa*. The wounds were treated with intravenous ceftazidime and cloxacillin.

During admission, the blister was surgically deroofed. The patient was later discharged with Seasorb Ag dressing. During follow-up, the wound was found to be filled with slough (Figure 5). She was re-admitted for treatment with maggot therapy. The ulcer healed completely after 2 weeks of maggot application (Figures 6 and 7).

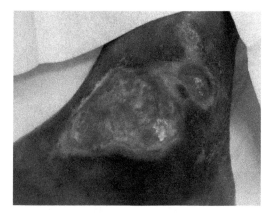

Figure 5:   Ulcer with Sloughy Wound Floor

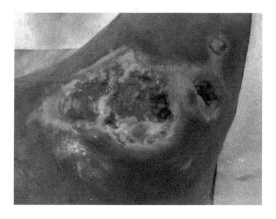

Figure 6:   Day 3 After Application of Maggots

Maggot therapy is potentially a good alternative to surgical debridement.[2] However, more evidence involving good randomised control studies is needed to show evidence that it is effective.

A good advantage of maggot therapy is that it can be carried out without the need for general or local anaesthesia. Patients with bad ulcers who are medically unfit to undergo general anaesthesia required for surgical debridement can undergo maggot therapy instead.

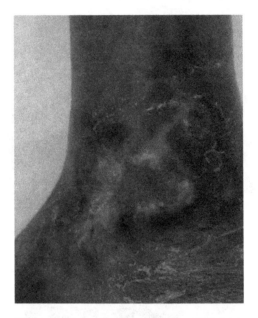

Figure 7:   Day 12 After Application of Maggots

A disadvantage of this treatment is that many patients are unable to psychologically accept the placement of maggots on their wounds.

References

1. Mexican Association for Wound Care and Healing, *Clinical Practice Guideline for the Treatment of Acute and Chronic Wounds with Maggot Debridement Therapy* (2010).
2. R.A. Sherman, Maggot therapy for treating diabetic foot ulcers unresponsive to conventional therapy, *Diabetes Care.* **B26B**(2): 446–451 (2003).

Chapter 27

Offloading Diabetic Foot

Aziz Nather

Introduction

The word "offload" means "to take away something unwanted" or "to get rid of something".

In the management of diabetic foot ulcer, "offloading" refers to relieving pressure from an ulcerated area. In an ulcer located in the weight-bearing portion of the foot, the ulcer will not heal unless offloading is achieved.

Offloading Devices

These include the following:

- specialised offloading shoes,
- offloading therapeutic insoles,
- total contact cast,
- Charcot restraint orthotic walker,
- Aircast,
- custom-made footwear.

Specialised Footwear

These include the following:

- ready-made diabetic shoe,
- forefoot wedge offloading shoe,
- heel wedge offloading shoe.

Ready-Made Diabetic Shoe

This specialised footwear is usually shoes which are very wide and have a soft and seamless inside lining (Figure 1). It is wide enough to accommodate a diabetic insole and bulky dressing for treating the ulcer. The insole and dressing would not be able to fit into normal shoes. An example is the "Gentle Step" shoe.

Offloading Insoles

Special therapeutic insoles are custom made to accommodate pressure areas and redistribute areas of high pressure (Figure 2). They are usually worn inside shoes. However, it could also be worn inside a walker to achieve ultimate wound healing.

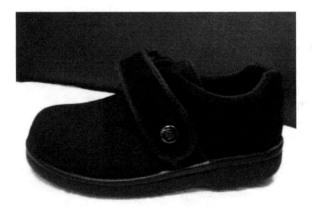

Figure 1:   Ready-made Diabetic Shoe with Soft Tissue Lining

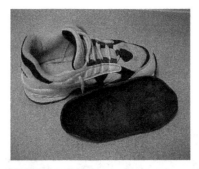

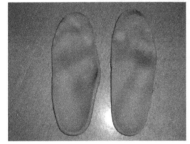
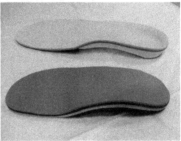

Figure 2:   Therapeutic Insoles

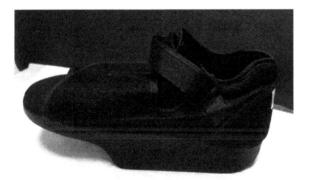

Figure 3:   Forefoot Wedge Offloading Shoe

Forefoot Wedge Offloading Shoe

This is special footwear to offload the forefoot area when walking
(Figure 3). It is used for ulcers on forefoot areas. It should only be worn
on one foot.

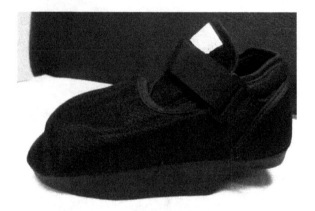

Figure 4:   Heel Wedge Offloading Shoe

Heel Wedge Offloading Shoe

This is another type of special footwear to offload the heel (Figure 4). It is useful for treatment of a heel ulcer. This should also be worn only on one side.

Charcot Joint Disease (CJD) and Offloading

The mainstay of treatment of CJD is non-operative offloading with Total Contact Cast (TCC) in the acute phase of the disease. TCC is the gold standard for offloading.

TCC is designed to conform to exact shape of the deformed foot. It distributes the weight and pressure over the entire sole. This allows the ulcer to heal by offloading the pressure area. It also achieves rapid reduction of oedema and reduces limb volume.

Figure 5 shows the application of TCC. This requires a skilled and experienced plaster technician. This is often the biggest limiting factor in the use of TCC.

A short below-knee plaster or fibreglass non-weight bearing cast is applied for acute CJD in a patient without an ulcer or in a patient with a non-infected ulcer. Non-weight bearing is obtained with the use of crutches.

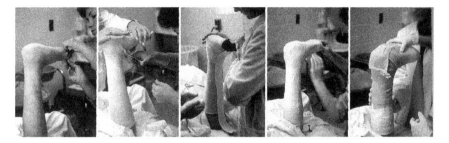

Figure 5: Application of Total Contact Cast

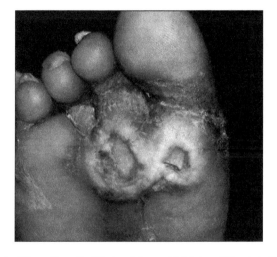

Figure 6: Plantar Ulcers Over the First and Second Metatarsal Heads in Patient with CJD

The plaster is changed every 2 weeks to allow inspection of the wound and to perform wound debridement if needed (Figure 6).

Non-weight bearing is recommended for a minimum period of 3–4 months for the acute phase of CJD. While total non-weight bearing is ideal for this treatment, compliance is often very poor.

Following NWB TCC for 3–4 months, an additional period of protected weight bearing is required with special shoes for at least 1–2 years, the period taken for the healing process of CJD to complete.

Offloading Walking Devices

Where there is poor compliance by patient to TTC or where skill to apply TTC is absent, other offloading devices could be used. These include the Charcot Restraint Orthotic Walker (CROW),[1] a pneumatic walking brace with a double metal upright AFO. The Aircast or ankle foot orthosis (Figure 7) containing a pneumatic envelope which is inflated to ensure a precise fit is also a suitable alternative offloading device. The ability of the patient to easily remove these devices means that the patients may not wear them. To ensure compliance, the removable cast walker can be rolled with a plaster or fibreglass cast roll (Figure 8). Such walking devices should be worn for at least 6 months.

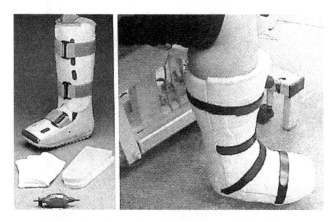

Figure 7:   Aircast Containing Pneumatic Envelope

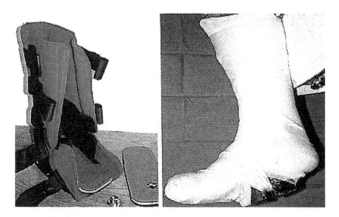

Figure 8:   Wrapping the Removable Walker with a Fibreglass Cast Roll

Custom-made Footwear

In general, following NWB TCC for 3–4 months or alternatively following offloading waling devices for 6 months or more, further protection is required for an additional period of 1–2 years using custom-made footwear. These therapeutic shoes are made with full-length inserts, rigid insoles, and a plastic or metal shank.[2] Plastazote inserts can also be used for insensate feet.

References

1. J.A. Mehta, C. Brown, and N. Sargeant, Charcot restraint orthotic walker, *Foot Ankle Int.* **19**: 619–623 (1998).
2. J.M. Giurini, Application and use of in-shoe orthoses in the conservative management of Charcot foot deformities, *Clin Podiatr Med Surg.* **11**: 271–278 (1994).

Chapter 28

Footwear and Offloading for Diabetic Foot Persons

Gulapar Srisawasdi

Introduction

Long-term diabetic persons especially those who do not have good control of blood sugar level will develop two major complications related to the feet: peripheral polyneuropathy and peripheral arterial occlusive disease.

Peripheral polyneuropathy is a microcirculation complication. It causes damage on peripheral sensory, motor, and autonomic nerves which occurs in feet first. Diabetic peripheral polyneuropathy is usually an irreversible process. It can start with painful neuropathy. However, the pathology ends up with insensate feet, intrinsic foot muscle atrophy, foot deformity, and dry and fragile skin. Unrecognised neuropathic foot ulcer easily develops due to abnormal plantar pressure distribution with repetitive trauma, especially over bony prominence areas.

Peripheral arterial occlusive disease is a macrocirculation complication. Large arteries in lower extremities become stenosis and finally occlude. Toes are the most affected part starting with ischemia, gangrene, and later on, ischemic foot ulcer develop.

Unfortunately, diabetic persons usually have both complications which makes it more complicated. Diabetes also causes poor immunity. Neuroischemic foot ulcer can easily get infected and most of the time ends up with amputation. Report on global amputation situation from the

International Working Group on the Diabetic Foot (IWGDF) showed that it is a serious problem. Every 20 seconds, a leg is lost due to diabetes.[1]

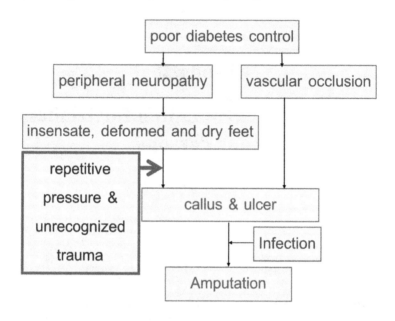

Definition of Footwear

Footwear is something we put on our feet. The expected benefits of footwear include foot protection, comfort, and improved health and functional performance. And most of all it has to be esthetic. Footwear does not mean only shoes but also insoles, foot orthosis, and socks.

Facts About Load on Foot

Feet are the foundation of our body. We use feet in every motion, even lying down in order to balance ourselves in all positions. Our feet bear a lot of weight. During standing barefoot, average loads on plantar pressure distribution over heel are about 60%, midfoot about 8%, forefoot about 28%, and toes about 4% of body weight.

During walking, the peak vertical forces are about 120% of body weight. And during running, the peak vertical forces could be up to 275% of body weight.

DM Foot Cycle and Roles of Offloading Footwear

Diabetic persons who have diabetic foot complications usually develop unrecognised foot ulcer and end up with amputation. The rate of recurrent ulcer is high, thus the rate of re-amputation at a higher level is also high. It was reported that about 40% of healed diabetic foot ulcer patients have recurrence within a year and up to 60% in 3 years.[2] The amputation on contralateral limb is not uncommon. Moreover, mortality rate after the first amputation is quite significant.

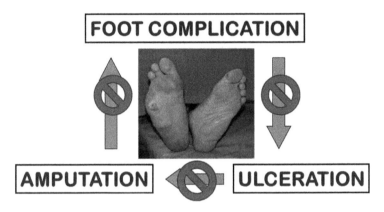

Neuropathic ulcer is more common than ischemic ulcer. Peripheral polyneuropathy causes imbalance between intrinsic and extrinsic foot muscles. The foot becomes deformed and insensate. The common neuropathic foot deformity in diabetes is claw toes which results in abnormal plantar pressure distribution. And the major cause of neuropathic ulcer is abnormal plantar pressure distribution. Skin breaks down after repetition of loads over bony prominence areas of insensate feet. Offloading footwear can play significant role in preventing ulcer development and helping ulcer healing. So, it can help end avoidable lower limb amputation.

2019 IWGDF Guideline for Prevention and Offloading Footwear

For diabetic persons who lost protective sensation in their feet, wearing improper footwear and walking barefoot or in thin-soled slippers are major causes of foot ulceration. These patients need to be concerned about appropriate footwear.

Proper footwear should be prescribed for at-risk feet in order to prevent ulceration. An important pre-ulcerative sign is callus. Callus is a toughened area of skin which has become thick and hard in response to repeated friction, pressure, or other irritation. Hard callus can cause skin and soft tissue underneath to break down. When a foot deformity or a pre-ulcerative sign is present, patients should be prescribed therapeutic shoes and custom-made foot/toe orthoses. Prescription of therapeutic footwear should demonstrate relieving enough plantar pressure while walking. It is recommended to keep plantar pressure below 200 kPa. In case of plantar foot ulcer, conventional or standard therapeutic shoes are not recommended.

The 2019 IWGDF offloading guideline[3] to heal diabetic neuropathic foot ulcer recommended line of approach by dividing ulcer into three groups: plantar forefoot or midfoot ulcer, plantar heel ulcer, and non-plantar ulcer.

1. *Plantar forefoot or midfoot ulcer*
   - No infection or ischemia
     1st line: None-removable knee-high offloading devices.
     2nd line: Removable knee-high offloading devices and encourage patient to wear.
     3rd line: Removable ankle-high offloading devices and encourage patient to wear.
     4th line: Felted foam with proper fitting shoes.
     5th line: Surgical offloading.
   - Infection and/or ischemia present
     Either mild infection or mild ischemia: Non-removable knee-high offloading devices.
     Both mild infection and mild ischemia or either moderate infection or moderate ischemia: Removable knee-high offloading devices and encourage patient to wear.
     Both moderate infection and moderate ischemia or either severe infection or severe ischemia: Address infection and/or ischemia. Offloading device based on patient's function, activity, and ambulatory status.
2. *Plantar heel ulcer*: Knee-high offloading device.

3. *Non-plantar ulcer*: Removable ankle-high offloading device, footwear modifications, toe spacers, or orthoses depending on type and location of ulcer.

Offloading Modalities

Total Contact Cast

Many literature supports the use of total contact cast to heal plantar foot ulcer. It helps in weight distribution by increasing contact area by 15–24%. This results in decreasing average pressure by 40–80% thus decreasing healing time. Technicians who work with the total contact cast need to be specially trained. Otherwise, it can cause a new ulcer.

Ankle Foot Orthosis (AFO)

The common AFO prescription for healing of diabetic foot ulcer includes Patella Tendon Bearing (PTB) AFO and Charcot Restraint Orthotic Walker (CROW).

Prefabricated Knee-high Device with an Appropriate Foot-device Interface

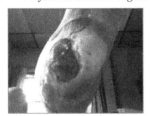
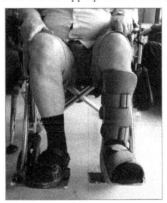

Patella Tendon Bearing AFO

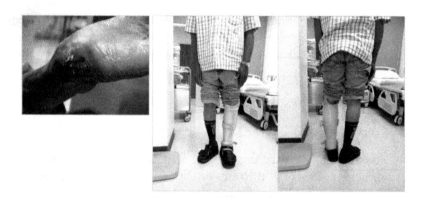

Common Foot Orthosis for Diabetic Foot Patients

Total contact orthosis is the recommended foot orthosis for diabetic foot patients. The orthosis is custom made to get the most contact area on the plantar surface of each individual's foot. Its functions include the following: weight distribution, shock absorption, decreased shearing force, protect pathologic area, and limit motion of affected joint. With all of these benefits, it helps in ulcer prevention and ulcer healing. However, it will provide the best result with proper shoes.

Total Contact Orthosis

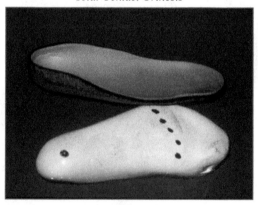

Common Shoe Modification for Diabetic Foot Patients

Rocker bottom sole is a common modification prescribed for diabetic foot patients. Its functions include the following: relieve pressure at specific area, replace motion of affected joints, improve gait, and decrease shock. There are five different types of rocker bottom modification. Toe only, severe angle, and negative heel modifications help offloading of the forefoot area. Heel to toe modification helps offloading of both the forefoot and hindfoot areas. And double rocker modification helps offloading of the midfoot area.

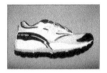 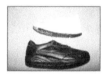 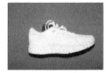 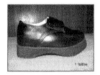

Custom Moulded Shoes

Custom moulded shoes will be prescribed for patients who have severe deformity that shoe modifications cannot be used to accommodate the deformity.

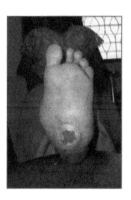 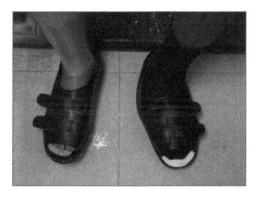

Shoes for Diabetic Foot Patients

Characteristics of Proper Shoes

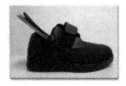 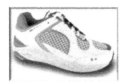 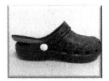

- **Design:** Toe areas should be covered since toes are the most common area for diabetic foot ulcer.
- **Outsole:** There should be built-in rocker bottom, especially at the forefoot area.
- **Midsole:** Material selected for midsole should provide the same cushioning properties as running shoes.
- **Insole:** Full-length removable insole is recommended with extra 3/16" or 5 mm thickness (depth shoes).
- **Materials:** Stretchable material is recommended in order to accommodate foot deformity. And it should have a good ventilation property as well.
- **Shoe closure:** Lace or Velcro-type closures are recommended to make it possible to adjust to volume changes throughout the day.

Characteristics of Improper Shoes

- Shoes that are made from vinyl or plastic.
- Thong sandals which can cause rubbing ulcer between toes.
- Pointed toe shoes which can cause ulcer on medial and lateral sides of big toe and fifth toe, respectively.
- High heel shoes which increase plantar pressure under forefoot area.

Proper Shoes Fit

Just having proper shoes is not enough to prevent ulceration. Diabetic persons with neuropathy tend to wear too tight shoes because they can feel only deep pressure. Since patients lose their sensation, they need to get education on proper shoes and how to select shoes. For high-risk group, fitting footwear is an important role of diabetic foot care personnel. Always evaluate the fit with the patient in the standing position. Foot size can increase by half a size or even one full size with weight-bearing position.

10 Tips to a Great Shoe Fit

1. There is no standard in shoe size even within the same brand. Do not buy shoes by size of the previous pairs. And do not ask anyone to buy shoes for you.
2. Both feet are not equal and change over time. Have both feet measured every time you purchase a pair of shoes.
3. Select shoes that match the shape of the feet. Do not try to squeeze feet to match the shape of the shoes.
4. When you shop for shoes, try on various types and styles. And select the most comfortable one.
5. Foot size can increase depending on activities and temperature each day. There should be 3/8–1/2 inch between the end of the longest toe and the end of the shoe.
6. Make sure the widest part of the foot fits the widest part of the shoe (across ball of foot).
7. Heels should fit. Some heel slippage can be allowed but should not create any scratch on skin.
8. Insole or orthosis affects the way a shoe fits. Put them in shoes before checking fitting.
9. Choose shoes appropriate for the activity and the time you perform that activity. Foot size changes depending on activities and temperature each day.
10. Finally, walk in the shoes to make sure it feels comfortable.

Socks

Diabetic persons should be advised to wear socks at all times. A common misunderstanding about socks that needs to be addressed to all patients is that socks cannot help in adjusting plantar pressure distribution. So, it cannot be used as offloading footwear. Proven benefits of socks include the following: preventing the frequency and severity of friction blisters, wick moisture away from feet, and reduce swelling in the feet and legs.

Currently, there are advanced technologies in garment manufacturing. New materials and techniques have been discovered. In terms of hydrophilic ranking, cotton is the leader, followed by wool, acrylic, and polypropylene, respectively. However, in terms of wicking moisture ranking, acrylic is the leader, followed by polypropylene, wool, and cotton respectively. Moreover, cotton becomes abrasive after multiple wash-wear cycles.

Risk Category and Recommending Footwear

Recommendation from the IWGDF suggests instructing an at-risk patient with diabetes to wear properly fitting footwear to prevent a foot ulcer.

Risk Category	Footwear
0 No LOPS and No PAD	Off-the-shelf footwear
1 LOPS or PAD	Must take extra care when selecting or being fitted with footwear
2 LOPS + PAD, or LOPS + foot deformity or PAD + foot deformity	Therapeutic footwear
3 LOPS or PAD, and one or more of the following: • history of a foot ulcer • a lower-extremity amputation (minor or major) • end-stage renal disease	

Notes: LOPS — Loss of protective sensation; PAD — peripheral arterial disease.

Conclusion

* Footwear for offloading is a well-accepted concept to promote ulcer healing and to prevent recurrent ulcer.
* Footwear management with proper fitting plays an important role in offloading.
* Proper ulcer care along with proper footwear are the keys to heal and prevent ulcer.
* Multidisciplinary approach is the most important. And patients need to be part of the team.

References

1. J.J. van Netten *et al.*, Prevention of foot ulcers in the at-risk patients with diabetes: a systematic review, *Diabet Metab Res Rev.* [online] **32**(1): 84–95 (2016).
2. Z.H. Huang, S.Q. Li, Y. Kou, L. Huang, T. Yu, and A. Hu, Risk factors for the recurrence of diabetic foot ulcers among diabetic patients: a meta-analysis, *Int Wound J.* **16**: 1373–1382 (2019).
3. S.A. Bus, D.G. Armstrong, C. Gooday, G. Jarl, C. Caravaggi, V. Viswanathan, and P.A. Lazzarini, Guidelines on offloading foot ulcers in persons with diabetes (IWGDF 2019 update), *Diabet Metab Res Rev.* 36(S1): 3269–3274 (2020).

Chapter 29

A Quick Look into Hyperbaric Oxygen Therapy

Aziz Nather

Introduction

Wounds need oxygen to heal. Hyperbaric Oxygen Therapy (HBOT) can play an important role as a complementary therapy for wound healing.

In chronic wounds, the tissue has become hypoxic. Hypoxia hinders wound healing. HBOT can increase the amount of oxygen reaching the tissue and thereby promote wound healing.

Hyperbaric Oxygen Therapy

HBOT is the inhalation of 100% oxygen at an atmospheric pressure greater than sea level — 2–3 times atmospheric pressure in a treatment chamber. This is carried out in a mono-place (Figure 1) or a multi-place chamber (Figures 2 and 3). The treatment of non-healing wound typically requires 20–30 HBOT sessions.

Effects of HBOT on Wound Healing

- *It increases tissue oxygen level* to support hypoxic tissue.
- *It reduces oedema.* The increase in blood oxygen concentration causes vasoconstriction which reduces oedema. This increases the rate of entry of oxygen into the tissues.

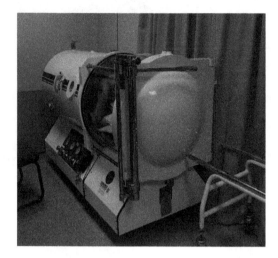

Figure 1:   Diagonal View of a Mono-place Hyperbaric Oxygen Chamber at Tan Tock Seng Hospital (TTSH)

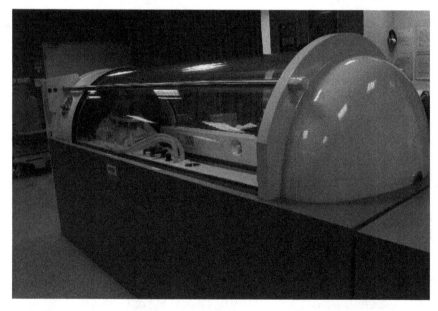

Figure 2:   Diagonal View of a 3-person Hyperbaric Oxygen Chamber at TTSH

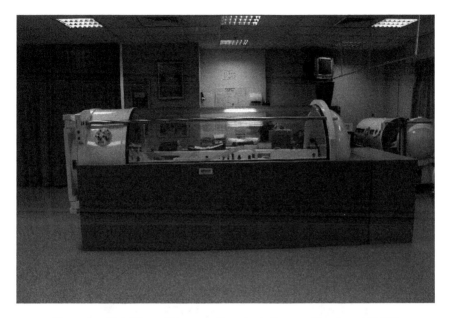

Figure 3:   Side View of 3-person Hyperbaric Oxygen Chamber at TTSH

- *It promotes tissue growth and repair:*
  o   it stimulates fibroblasts to synthesise collagen
  o   it stimulates the release of cytokines and growth factors
- *It combats infection:*
  o   it activates neutrophils
  o   it enhances phagocytosis
  o   it inhibits bacterial growth
  o   it inhibits release of bacterial endotoxins
  o   it improves effect of antibiotics

Case Study

A 67-year-old Chinese lady with type 2 diabetes of 7 years duration with infected bilateral wet gangrene of all toes (Figure 4) with purulent discharge for one month. Both dorsalis pedis and posterior tibial pulses were not palpable. In the right foot, ABI was 0.4 and TBI 0.2. In the left foot, ABI was 0.8 and TBI 0.55.

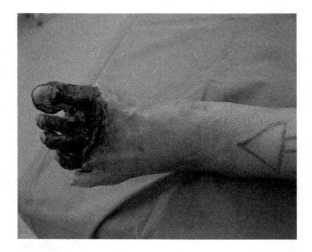

Figure 4:   Wet Gangrene Toes in Left Foot

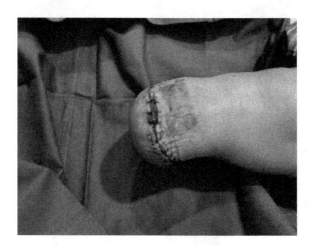

Figure 5:   Right Below-Knee Amputation Stump 18th Post-operative Day

Below-knee amputation was done on the right side (Figure 5) and a Pirogoff amputation on the left (Figure 6).

Since vascularity was borderline, the patient was sent for HBOT and completed a course of 30 sessions. Both wounds have healed successfully (Figures 5 and 6).

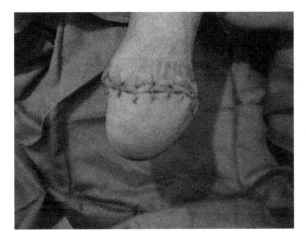

Figure 6: Left Pirogoff Amputation Stump 13th Post-operative Day

Normobaric Oxygen Challenge Test

Transcutaneous Oxymetry (TcPo) is a simple, non-invasive tool to measure peri-wound oxygenation and microcirculatory blood flow. It is useful to provide an indication of the potential benefit of HBOT in wound healing.

Take a TcPo measurement at sea level −1 atmospheric pressure with the patient breathing air. Repeat the measurement with the patient inhaling 100% oxygen:

- If TcPo level remains <35 mmHg or if increase in TcPo level remains, 10 mmHg 90% of patients will fail to heal with HBOT.
- If TcPo level increases >100 mmHg, 90% of patients will be successful in wound healing.

HBOT and Necrotising Fasciitis

In necrotising fasciitis, the key treatment is radical surgical debridement coupled with an intravenous antibiotic regime for necrotising fasciitis protocol. However, when possible, HBOT is a useful adjunct to promote healing.

HBOT and Microangiopathy

While in most cases vasculopathy in diabetic foot is due to peripheral arterial disease due to atherosclerosis involving medium-sized arteries, in some cases, it is due to microangiopathy involving small vessels — the terminal arterioles.

Macroangiopathy can be treated by revascularisation — angioplasty or bypass performed by the vascular surgeon. In contrast, microangiopathy cannot be treated by revascularisation. The only treatment option available is by HBOT which increases the tissue oxygen level directly to promote wound healing and avoid minor or distal amputation.

HBOT or no HBOT? — The Continuing Controversy

Kranke et al.[1] in a *Cochrane Review* showed that HBOT significantly improved wound healing in the short term but not long term. However, they found no difference in amputation.

Meta-analysis by Brouwer et al.[2] found that HBOT reduces major amputation but was ineffective in wound healing. Meta-analysis by Sharma et al.[3] also showed similar results to that by Brouwer. They found no effect on the reduction of minor amputation rate.

Until more evidence is available, the role of HBOT remains controversial.

References

1. P. Kranke et al., Hyperbaric oxygen therapy for chronic wounds, *Cochrane Database Syst Rev.* (2015).
2. R.J. Brouwer et al., A systematic review and meta-analysis of hyperbaric oxygen therapy for diabetic foot ulcers with arterial insufficiency, *J Vasc Surg.* 71(2): 682–692 (2020).
3. R. Sharma et al., Efficacy of hyperbaric oxygen therapy for diabetic foot ulcer, a systematic review and meta-analysis of controlled clinical trials, *Nat Portfolio Sci Rep.* (2021).

Chapter 30

Charcot Joint Disease

Aziz Nather

Introduction

Charcot Joint Disease (CJD) or neuropathic joint is a musculoskeletal condition characterised by damage and disruption of joints and their surrounding bones. Its pathology starts from the loss of protective sensation and this leads to gradual damage and disruption of joints and their adjacent bones. CJD occurs most commonly in the foot and ankle.

Historical Background

In 1868, Jean-Martin Charcot,[1] a French neurologist, gave the first detailed description of the neuropathic aspect of CJD. In 1936, William Riley Jordan[2] described the association between neuropathic arthropathy and diabetes mellitus. He attributed a typical painless Charcot joint of the ankle in an elderly woman with diabetes to be "a diabetic process of a neurologic trophic nature". Since then, diabetes has been found to be the leading cause of CJD.

Epidemiology and Etiology

CJD may occur bilaterally (Figure 1). It is associated with a longstanding duration of diabetes and peripheral neuropathy. In the early stages, CJD is

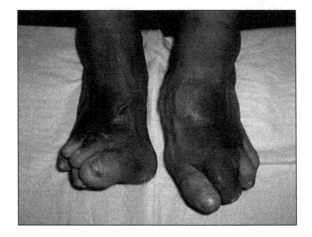

Figure 1:   Severe Deformity of Forefoot, Medial Convexity of Mid-foot, Left Ankle Deformity, and Distended Veins in a Patient with Bilateral CJD

characterised by acute inflammation which eventually leads to bone and joint fracture, dislocation, instability, and gross deformity.[3]

Pathogenesis

Three major theories exist regarding the pathophysiology of Charcot arthropathy:

- Neurotraumatic Theory (German)
- Neurovascular Theory (French)
- Modern Theory

While peripheral neuropathy develops over decades, the progression of Charcot foot can occur in a matter of weeks or months initiated by a minor trauma, such as twisting of the foot.

Neurotraumatic Theory

Charcot believed that the development of enlarged joints was initiated by "spontaneous fracture". Johnson[4] explained further that a stress fracture caused by microtrauma in an insensate foot could go undetected due to loss of peripheral sensation and proprioception. The patient continues to traumatise the bone and soft tissues, leading to hyperemia. Inadequate protection causes impaired recovery and healing. A vicious cycle arises due to continuous microtrauma and impairment of the repair responses. This eventually leads to Charcot joint destruction.[5]

Neurovascular Theory

The neurovascular theory suggests that a dysregulated autonomic nervous system causes the extremities to receive increased blood flow. This in turn leads to a mismatch in bone destruction and synthesis, resulting in osteopenia. The atrophic and osteopenic bone easily becomes traumatised.

Modern Theory

The modern theory attributed the Charcot process to the cytokines released.

Medical History

The diagnosis of CJD is often based on clinical features. These include profound unilateral swelling, increased skin temperature (by 3–7°C), erythema, joint effusion, and foot and ankle deformity in an insensate extremity. Concomitant ulceration is common. It may be difficult to distinguish from osteomyelitis. As the disease progresses, deformity appears. The longitudinal and transverse arches of foot may collapse, resulting in a rocker bottom foot.

Clinical Phases of CJD

CJD clinically presents in three phases:

- Acute Charcot Arthropathy
- Bone Destruction/Deformity Phase
- Stabilisation Phase

Acute Phase

The acute phase presents with unilateral swelling, erythema, increase in local skin temperature, bounding pulses, prominent veins, and joint effusion. In CJD, prominent veins are caused by venous shunting. Pain or discomfort may be minimal due to underlying neuropathy. Patients usually have a recent foot or ankle injury with swelling but minimal pain.

Bone Destruction/Deformity Phase

In this phase, the foot is swollen and warm. Collapse of the medial arch of the foot becomes more apparent. Progression of deformity results in a rocker-bottom foot.

　　This phase presents radiological findings of bone fragmentation, new bone formation, subluxation, and dislocation. It occurs within weeks of the onset of this condition. The involvement of tarsometatarsal joints leads to broadening of the mid-foot, giving rise to a medial convexity. The involvement of the metatarsophalangeal and inter-phalangeal joints together with imbalance of the muscles in the feet leads to toe deformities e.g. claw toes (Figure 2). The tips of the toes are prone to ulceration. The foot becomes unstable and requires some form of immobilisation.

Stabilisation Phase

In this phase, the foot is no longer red or swollen. The deformity may be marked, but the patients are asymptomatic. Bone integrity is strengthened and the involved joints develop into pseudoarthroses or become fused.

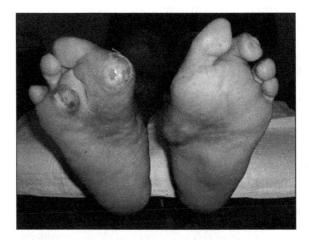

Figure 2:　Clawing and Overriding of Toes with Medial Convexity of Left Mid-foot. Callosities Present Over Right First and Fourth Metatarsal Heads

Radiological Presentation

Radiographically, CJD can present in two different ways:

Atrophic

Atrophic patterns have the characteristic dissolution of bone and joint surfaces, commonly seen in the more lateral metatarsal regions.

Hypertrophic

The hypertrophic pattern is more common and can present anywhere within the foot. The radiographic features — 6 Ds of hypertrophy[6] — are increased **D**ensity (subchondral sclerosis), **D**estruction of bone, **D**ebris (intra-articular loose bodies) production, **D**islocation, **D**istention of joint, and **D**isorganisation.

Eichenholtz Classification System

The hypertrophic pattern of CJD is typically defined according to the Eichenholtz classification system.[7] It is based on radiographic appearance as well as physiologic stages of the process. This classification system is useful to determine the patient's prognosis and to gauge the optimal timing for arthrodesis. Surgical intervention is most effective when it is performed in early stage 1 or late stage 3 disease.

Stage 0: At Risk Stage — The "Charcot in Situ" Stage

In this stage, there is no radiographic change in bone — the *"Charcot in situ" Stage*.

Stage 1: Developmental Stage — Acute Stage

In the acute stage, hyperemia due to autonomic neuropathy weakens bones and ligaments. This leads to diffuse swelling, joint laxity, subluxation, and frank dislocation. The patient presents with an acute inflammatory process. Bone fragmentation and joint disruption are visible in radiographs (Figure 3), with osseous debris surrounding the affected joint

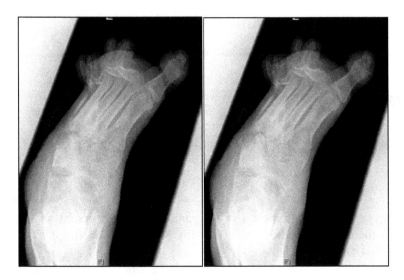

Figure 3:   Plain Radiographs Showing Visible Joint Disruption and Bony Fragmentation Involving Fore-foot and Mid-foot (Developmental Phase)

Stage 2: Coalescent (Quiescent) Stage

In the coalescent or quiescent phase, the osseous debris is resorbed and the larger fragments fuse together. There is a decrease in warmth, redness, and swelling. Radiographs show sclerotic bone surrounding the joint, callus formation, and fusion of larger bony fragments.

Stage 3: Remodeling Stage

Bone integrity is strengthened. The joints are re-established either as pseudoarthroses or actual fusions. Radiographs show remodelling of bone or bony ankylosis. The foot becomes stable but deformed. This phase last months to years.

Brodsky's System of Classification

Brodsky's system of classification[8] is based on anatomic location.

Type 1: Tarsometatarsal (Lisfranc's) joints

Approximately 60% of cases are Type 1. Residual deformity in this area with collapse of the longitudinal arch produces the rocker-bottom foot deformity. Ulcer often develops in the sole at the apex of this deformity.

Type 2: Hindfoot

This involves the subtalar, talonavicular, and calcaneocuboid joints. It is the second most common site — about 20% of cases.

Type 3

(a) Ankle Joint
(b) Posterior Calcaneus

Type 3 occurs mainly in the ankle and accounts for 10% of cases.

Type 4: Multiple Regions

Each region may be at a different Eichenholtz stage.

Type 5: Forefoot

Type 5 is uncommon.

Clinical Examination

A high index of clinical suspicion is required to diagnose CJD in a patient with a swollen or deformed foot, especially when neuropathy is present. A complete physical examination must include neurological and vascular examination. Neurological examination includes pinprick, position sense, and vibration sense with a tuning fork. In addition, assessment of vibration sensation (with a biothesiometer) and touch sensation (with 5.07 Semmes–Weinstein monofilament) are useful tests for diagnosis. The risk of developing a neuropathic ulcer is much higher if the biothesiometer reading is greater than 26 volts.

Investigations

Hematological and Biochemical Studies

Blood tests performed include full blood count, serum urea, and electrolytes. White blood cell counts are not raised except when infection is present. C-reactive Protein (CRP) levels and Erythrocyte Sedimentation Rate (ESR) are also raised with superimposed infection.

Tissue Biopsy

Tissue biopsy is the most specific method (gold standard) for diagnosing CJD. A definitive diagnosis of CJD can be made with a synovial tissue biopsy, which will show shards of bone and cartilage embedded within the synovium.[9]

Radiographs

Radiographs performed include weight-bearing anteroposterior, lateral, and oblique views of the foot or anteroposterior and lateral views of the ankle. Radiographs provide valuable information as to the anatomic location of the disease involvement as well as the phase the disease process is in.

Conservative Treatment of CJD

The treatment of CJD is mainly non-operative. Treatment depends on the phase of CJD.

Acute Phase

In this phase, early immobilisation and offloading are critical.

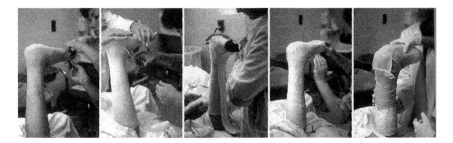

Figure 4:   Application of a Total Contact Cast

Offloading with Total Contact Cast

The affected lower extremity is immobilised in a short, below-knee, plaster or fibreglass, non-weight bearing Total Contact Cast (TCC) (Figure 4). Complete non-weight weight bearing is achieved with the use of crutches. This is recommended for a minimum period of 3–4 months. However, compliance is usually poor.

TCC is the gold standard for offloading. It is designed to conform exactly to the shape of the affected foot and ankle. It distributes weight and pressure over the entire plantar aspect of the foot. The offloading provided allows the ulcer to heal by relieving the bony prominent area from excessive pressure. It also reduces oedema rapidly and causes the limb volume to decrease.

The cast must be changed at regular intervals of 1–2 weeks to evaluate the foot. Patients with insensitive feet may develop sores in the cast. The ulcer present is inspected at regular intervals for change of dressing and the wound is debrided if needed.

Offloading with Walking Devices

In patients who refuse to comply with TCC or in situations where expertise is lacking to apply TCC by an experienced plaster technician, alternative offloading walking devices may be used. These include the Charcot Restraint Orthotic Walker (CROW),[10] a pneumatic walking brace with a double metal upright ankle foot orthosis or the Aircast (Figure 5) with a pneumatic envelope inflated to ensure a precise fit.

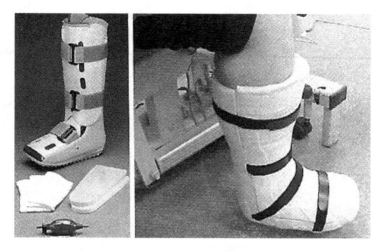

Figure 5: Aircast Containing a Pneumatic Envelope

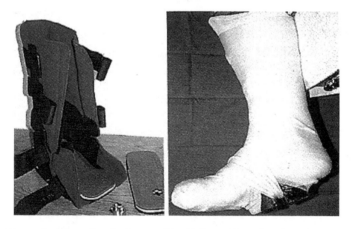

Figure 6: Wrapping the Removable Walker with a Fibreglass Cast Roll

To improve compliance, these walking devices can be made non-removable by applying a fibreglass cast roll around the body of the walker (Figure 6). Such a walking device should be worn for at least 6 months.

Custom-made Footwear

Following a non-weight bearing TCC for 3–4 months, or following offloading walking devices for 6 months, further protection is required for an additional period of 1–2 years using custom-made footwear. These extra-depth shoes include full-length inserts, have rigid soles, and have a plastic or metal shank.[11] If an ulcer is present, a rocker-bottom sole can be used. In addition, Plastazote insert can be used for insensate feet.

Adjunctive Therapy

Bisphosphonates

Bisphosphonates, a potent inhibitor of bone resorption, may be used as adjunctive therapy to expedite the conversion of the acute process to the quiescent, reparative stage. Bisphosphonates inhibit the osteoclastic activity of bone breakdown. They also promote healing of bone. Jude *et al.*[12] found that a single intravenous infusion of the bisphosphonate, pamidronate, led to a reduction in bone breakdown in Charcot neuroarthropathy.

Operative Treatment of CJD

The main indications of surgery are ulceration of the foot and instability of joints. Infected ulcer is treated with drainage of abscess or debridement together with offloading to allow the ulcer to heal. Prophylactic foot surgery to correct bony deformity may be performed to prevent ulcer formation. In other situations, exostectomy of bony prominence is needed. Fusion of unstable joints is the other surgical treatment performed. In general, bony surgery is best avoided during the acute phase of CJD due to the hyperemia, osteopenia, and oedema present.

Outcome of Treatment

The outcome depends on when the diagnosis is made and treatment instituted. A more favourable outcome occurs when joints are treated within two weeks of injury and when there is strict adherence to weight-bearing precautions.

Location of the disease also affects the outcome. Forefoot osteoarthropathy heals faster than midfoot, hindfoot, or ankle arthropathy.

The extent of the injury to bone and soft tissue in CJD also affects healing time. The more severe the Charcot changes, the longer it takes to heal, and the greater the likelihood that it would develop a permanent deformity. In general, it takes 1–2 years for a Charcot Joint to heal.

References

1. J.M. Charcot, Sur quelaquestarthropathies qui paraissendependerd'une lesion du cerveauou de la moeleepiniere. *Arch Des Physiol Norm et Path.* **1**: 161–171 (1868).
2. W.R. Jordan, Neuritic manifestations in diabetes mellitus, *Arch Int Med.* **57**: 307–366 (1936).
3. B.M. Perrin *et al.*, Charcot osteoarthropathy of the foot, *Austr Family Phys.* **39**(3): 117–119 (2010)
4. J.T. Johnson, Neuropathic fractures and joint injuries, *J Bone Joint Surg.* **49(A)**: 1–30 (1967).
5. S. Meyer, The pathogenesis of diabetic Charcot joints, *The Iowa Ortho J.* **12**: 63–70 (1992).
6. T. Yochum and L. Rowe, Neuropathic arthropathy, *Yochum and Rowe's Essentials of Skeletal Radiology,* 2nd Edition, Baltimore, USA, William & Wilkins, pp. 842–849 (1987).
7. S.N. Eichenholz, in: C. Charles (ed.), *In Charcot Joints*, Thomas, Springfield, pp. 1–20 (1966).
8. J.W. Brodsky, The diabetic foot, in: M.J. Coughlin and R.A. Mann (eds.), *Surgery of the Foot and Ankle*, 7th Edition, St. Louis, MO, Mosby, pp. 895–969 (1999).
9. L. Lee, P. Blume, and B. Sumpio, CJD in diabetes mellitus, *Ann Vasc Surg.* **17**(5): 571–580 (2003).
10. J.A. Mehta, C. Brown, and N. Sargeant, Charcot restraint orthotic walker, *Foot Ankle Int.* **19**: 619–623 (1998).
11. J.M. Giurini, Applications and use of in-shoe orthoses in the conservative management of Charcot foot deformity, *Clin Podiatr Med Surg.* **11**: 271–278 (1994).
12. E.B. Jude, Bisphosphonates in the treatment of Charcot neuroarthropathy: a double-blind randomised controlled trial, *Diabetologia.* **44**: 2032–2037 (2001).

Chapter 31

Necrotising Fasciitis

Aziz Nather

Introduction

Necrotising fasciitis (NF) is an infection located in the deep fascia which results in necrosis (death and damage) of the subcutaneous tissues. It is one of the most dangerous conditions that could develop in a limb. NF causes severe infection that spreads rapidly and can be fatal. It is also commonly known as the "killer bug disease" or "flesh-eating bacterial infection".

NF can be caused by various types of bacteria and fungi. The infection can be a result of a single pathogen or can be polymicrobial. The bacterial group A beta-haemolytic streptococci (*Streptococcus pyogenes*) is the most common cause of NF.

Given the rapid progression of the disease, patients with NF should be treated as an emergency. However, NF can be difficult to diagnose in its early stage. A high index of suspicion is important. Once the infection reaches the connective tissue, the spread can be so fast that it can get out of control, even with both antibiotics and debridement surgery. In certain cases, the spread can be so fast that it may be fatal within 48 hours.

Types of Necrotising Fasciitis

The types of NF are as follows:

- Type I
  - Polymicrobial NF

- ■ Can be mistaken for a simple wound cellulitis
- ■ Usually occurs after a trauma or surgery
- Type II
  - ■ Group A streptococcal NF
  - ■ Known as the "flesh-eating" bacterial infection

History

Profile of Patients

NF is not uncommon in Singapore. Wong *et al.*[1] reported 89 patients in Changi General Hospital alone over a 7-year period from January 1997 to August 2002. The mean age of patients with NF was found to be about 56 years.

Predisposing Factors

NF is common in immunocompromised patients. These include patients with diabetes, cancer, alcoholism, vascular insufficiency (impaired blood flow), organ transplants, and HIV.

Comorbidities

Comorbidities are common in patients with NF. Wong *et al.*[1] found diabetes mellitus to be the most common comorbidity, present in 70.8% of patients, peripheral vascular disease in 22.5%, chronic liver disease in 3.4%, and cancer in 2.2%.

Liu *et al.*[2] in a study of 87 consecutive patients of NF from 1999 to 2004 also found diabetes mellitus to be the most common comorbidity: 53.2%.

History

NF can develop following trauma, around foreign bodies in surgical wounds or after surgical procedures including cardiac catheterisation. Idiopathic cases can also be present.

Pathophysiology

Bacteria spread from the subcutaneous tissue along the superficial and deep fascial planes. The bacterial enzymes and toxins they produce facilitate the rapid spread of the disease. Streptococcal pyrogenic exotoxins lead to the release of cytokines and produce clinical signs, such as hypotension. The poor prognosis in NF has been linked to infection with certain Streptococcal strains.

In NF, Group-A haemolytic Streptococci and Staphylococcus *aureus* alone or in synergism are frequently the initiating infecting bacteria. Other aerobic and anaerobic pathogens include Bacteroides, Peptostreptococcus, Enterobacteriaceae, Coliforms, Proteus, Pseudomonas, and Klebsiella.

Some cases of NF can be caused by Vibrio *vulnificus*. This organism is seen more often in patients with chronic liver dysfunction and often follows the consumption of raw seafood.

Wong *et al.*[1] found polymicrobial infection (NF Type I) to be the most common (53.9%) with Streptococci and Enterobacteriaceae being the most common pathogens. Group A Streptococcus was the most common pathogen of monomicrobial NF (Type II). They found diabetes mellitus to be the most common associated comorbidity (70.8%).

Examination

Clinical Findings

In the early phase, patients complain of severe pain out of proportion to their seemingly minor skin changes. He can also present with fever, chills, dehydration, and tachycardia. A detailed history of the patient should be taken to find out about any recent illness, injury, or exposure to seawater.

The patient's condition can deteriorate very quickly. After 1–2 days, there is an onset of severe pain, swelling, and erythema at the site of trauma or recent surgery. This is often mistaken for cellulitis, as the necrosis of the deep fascia under the skin is not visible. However, unlike cellulitis, tenderness extends beyond the site of infection.

After 2–4 days, the patient develops swelling of the skin. Other changes include skin ulceration, supra-lesional vesiculation or bullae formation (formation of blisters) (Figure 1), necrotic eschars (black

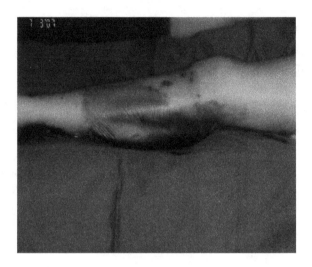

Figure 1:   Large Blister on the Medial Side of the Left Leg

scabs), and gas formation in the tissue. A dusky or purplish skin discolouration can be observed. Palpation can reveal crepitus (crackling or grating sounds under the skin) due to the formation of subcutaneous gas from the bacteria.

After 4–5 days, hypotension (low blood pressure) and septic shock (life-threateningly low blood pressure due to overwhelming infection) develop. Patients become confused, and if the NF is not kept under control, the results could be fatal.

Investigations

- **Blood Tests**
  A full blood count and urea/electrolytes should be performed. Pointers to NF[1] include the following:
  - o   C-reactive protein   >16   mg/dL
  - o   White cell count   >15 × 10^9/L
  - o   Haemoglobin   <13.5 g/dL
  - o   Sodium   <135 mmol/L
  - o   Creatinine   >141 μmol/L

- o   Glucose   >10   mmol/dL
- o   Creatine kinase   >600 U/L
- o   Urea   >18   mg/dL

Wong *et al.*[3] developed a novel diagnostic scoring system to distinguish NF from other soft tissue infections based on laboratory tests routinely performed for evaluation of soft tissue infections: the Laboratory Risk Indicator for Necrotising Fasciitis (LRINEC) score based on a study of 140 patients with NF and 309 patients with severe cellulitis or abscess in two institutions in Singapore. The six laboratory indicators were total white cell count, haemoglobin, sodium, glucose, serum creatinine, and C-reactive protein. Patients with an LRINEC score of more than 6 should be carefully evaluated for the presence of NF.

Microbiological Tests

Gram staining and culture should be conducted on blood cultures, exudates (fluid from the site of infection) by a wound swab and biopsied tissue. The results obtained can be useful in determining the organism(s) responsible for the infection. A fungal culture can also be obtained from patients who are immunocompromised and those who have a history of trauma.

Wong *et al.*[1] found polymicrobial synergistic infection to be the most common (53.9%), with Streptococci and Enterobacteriaceae being the most common pathogens identified. Group-A Streptococcus was the most common cause of monomicrobial NF.

Radiological Tests

Local radiographs can show the presence of gas in the subcutaneous fascial planes (Figure 2(a) and 2(b)). This is characteristic of NF. MRI scans can be used to indicate the extent of surgical debridement required. However, clinical signs showing severe tenderness at fascial level coupled with presence of gas on plain radiographs are sufficient to indicate the presence and extent of NF. Urgent preparations for surgery can be made without delay in waiting for time-consuming and costly MRI.

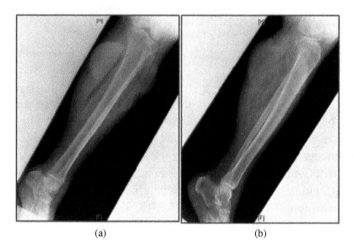

(a)   (b)

Figure 2:   (a) and (b) Gas Shadow Seen in the Calf of the Same Patient Shown in Figure 1

Bedside Finger Test

This is carried out under local anaesthesia. It involves probing the deep fascia with a gloved index finger through a 2-cm incision. Lack of bleeding, the presence of "dishwasher pus", and non-contracting muscles after the blunt finger dissection are indicative of NF.[4]

A family conference must be convened as soon as possible to inform the family of the seriousness of their condition — high mortality (between 20% and 25%) and severe morbidities which include hypotensive shock and acute renal shutdown. The need for urgent surgical debridement and post-operative care in an intensive care unit must be emphasised. The chances of a second debridement are high (about 50%) and further closure of the wound with split skin grafting might be needed. The immediate dressing of the operative wound with negative pressure dressing must also be explained. Finally, the risks of lower limb amputation (10–20%), if the debridement fails to debulk bacterial and toxic load, must also be informed.

Treatment

NF requires immediate and aggressive treatment immediately after its diagnosis. The patient should be hospitalised in an intensive care unit and his haemodynamic parameters should be closely monitored. Intravenous antibiotics must be started as soon as possible. Post-operatively, a peripherally inserted central catheter (PICC) line must be inserted.

Antibiotics

The following antibiotic regimes could be used, as they are usually recommended by the infectious disease consultant.

Combination Therapy

This approach involves the use of two or three antibiotics:

- Crystalline penicillin (e.g. 2–4 mega 8 hourly) plus clindamycin to cover aerobes (usually Gram-negative organisms).
- If the patient is allergic to penicillin, give meropenem plus clindamycin or.
- Clindamycin plus ciprofloxacin plus metronidazole.

  These are regimes based on UK hospital guidelines.[5]

NUH Antibiotics Guidelines

- IV benzylpenicillin + IV ceftazidime + IV clindamycin.[6]
- Treatment should be discussed with the local consultant microbiologist and should be adjusted once culture results have returned.
- For suspected Vibrio spp., include tetracycline and third-generation cephalosporin (e.g. doxycycline plus ceftazidime); ciprofloxacin may be an alternative.[6]

Medical Treatment

- Nutritional support is required from day one, owing to the high protein and fluid loss from the wound (similar to major burns). In severe cases, patients may need twice their basal calorie requirements. Nasogastric feeding may be helpful.
- Intravenous immunoglobulin may be a useful adjunct in severe Streptococcal infections (to neutralise Streptococcal toxins).
- Hyperbaric oxygen therapy for NF is controversial.[5]

Surgery

Surgical debridement must be performed as soon as possible for higher chances of survival. The first surgery is the most important. To ensure that the debridement is extensive, the surgical incisions should be deep and should extend beyond the areas of necrosis until viable tissue is reached. This ensures that no infected tissue is left behind. Debridement is best done through two incisions: one on the medial side of the limb and the other on the lateral side of the limb. All necrotic fat, unhealthy tissue, and necrotic fascia must be surgically excised. If the exposed underlying muscle is necrotic and non-viable, this must also be debrided until healthy, pink, contractile muscle is left behind (Figure 3).

A sample of tissue is sent for culture and sensitivity. The extensive wound is then flushed with hydrogen peroxide and with 2–3 L of normal saline using jet lavage. Haemostasis is carefully and meticulously secured. A vacuum dressing is then applied. The VAC dressings must be changed and the wound must be inspected every 2–3 days. If further pus, slough, or necrosis is seen, a second or even third debridement must be performed.

Once the infection markers are down, the wound culture is negative, and healthy granulation tissue is seen in the wound bed, a split skin grafting is performed (Figure 4).

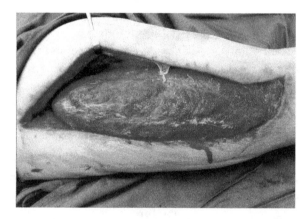

Figure 3:   Showing Sero-purrulent Fluid and Unhealthy Deep Fascia. Radical Debridement Done to Excise All Unhealthy Tissues in 54-Year-Old Chinese Diabetic Female with NF. VAC Dressing Applied. Second and Third Debridements Required Over Next 10 Days

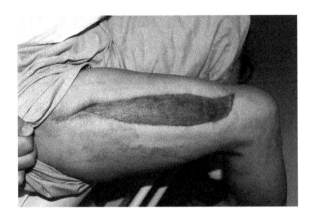

Figure 4:   Healed SSG on the Lateral Aspect of the Thigh in Same Patient Shown in Figure 3 One Month Later

In advanced cases of NF, an amputation may need to be performed due to the progression of the disease resulting in irreversible necrosis and gangrene. Lim *et al.*[7] showed that primary amputation should be considered in a patient with advanced NF. Amputation is done to completely remove the sepsis in the limb and reduces the need for repeated procedures involving general anaesthesia. This may be necessary for patients with multiple comorbidities including heart disease, as multiple operations place the patient under significant risk.

Complications

- NF carries a significant mortality rate, particularly if marine organisms (above) are involved.
- Septic or toxic shock (the latter due to streptococcal endotoxin production).
- The deep tissue infection may lead to vascular occlusion, ischaemia, and tissue necrosis. There may be nerve damage and muscle necrosis.
- Large areas of tissue loss may require skin grafting, flap surgery, or amputation.

In a study of 451 patients with NF involving both the upper and lower limb, Angoules *et al.*[8] found 22.3% underwent amputation or disarticulation of a limb following the failure of multiple debridements.

Mortality

The poor prognosis in NF has been linked to infection with certain Streptococcal strains. The mortality rate can be as high as 20–25%. Angoules et al.[8] found a mortality rate of 21.9%, while Shimizu and Tokuda[9] found it to be 25%.

Wong et al.[1] found that factors such as advanced age, two or more associated comorbidities, and a delay in surgery of more than 24 hours adversely affected the outcome. Multivariate analysis showed that a delay in surgery of more than 24 hours was correlated with increased mortality ($p < 0.05$; relative risk $= 9.4$). They concluded that early operative debridement must be done to reduce mortality.

A high index of suspicion is very important in view of the paucity of specific cutaneous findings in the early course of the disease. Liu et al.[2] found multivariate logistic regression analysis showed that factors such as thrombocytopenia (abnormally low amount of platelets), anaemia, two or more associated comorbidities, a delay of more than 24 hours from onset of symptoms to surgery, and age greater than 60 were independently associated with mortality.

References

1. C.H. Wong et al., Necrotizing fasciitis: clinical presentation, microbiology and determinants of mortality. *J Bone Joint Surg Am.* **85**: 1454–1460 (2003).
2. Y.M. Liu et al., Microbiology and factors affecting mortality in necrotizing fasciitis. *J Microbiol Immunol Infect.* **38**(6): 430–435 (2005).
3. C.H. Wong et al., The LRINEC (laboratory risk indicator for necrotizing fasciitis) score: a tool for distinguishing necrotizing fasciitis from other soft tissue infections. *Crit Care Med.* **32**(7): 1535–1541 (2004).
4. T.J. Andreasen et al., Massive infectious soft tissue injury: diagnosis and management of necrotising fasciitis and purpura fulminans. *Plast Reconstr Surg.* **107**(4): 1025–1035 (2001).
5. N. Hartree, Necrotising fasciitis, *Egton Medical Information Systems* (2011). Available from: https://www.patient.co.uk/doctor/Necrotising-Fasciitis.htm.
6. National University Hospital Guidelines (2019).
7. Y.J. Lim et al., Necrotising fasciitis and traditional medical therapy — dangerous liaison. *Ann Acad Med.* **35**: 270–273 (2006).
8. G. Angoules, Necrotising fasciitis of upper and lower limb: a systematic review. *Injury.* **38**(S5): S19–S26 (2007).
9. T. Shimizu and Y. Tokuda, Necrotising fasciitis. *Inter Med.* **49**: 1051–1057 (2010).

Chapter 32

Rehabilitating the Below-knee Amputee

Aziz Nather and Lim Kean Seng Andrew

Introduction

The loss of a limb can result in major disability and psychological trauma to the affected individual. An integrated comprehensive approach by an interdisciplinary team following limb amputation is paramount for successful surgical and functional outcome.

Two main goals of the management of limbs in the post-amputation, pre-prosthetic stage are obtaining maximal functional independence and optimising the residual limb for prosthesis fitting.[1]

Areas of focus would include the following:

- pain control,
- wound care and oedema control,
- contracture prevention and joint range of motion,
- physical conditioning,
- psychological support and education.

Pain Control

Pain can be from various sources. It is important to distinguish phantom pain from that of a surgical wound. Phantom pain is characterised as intermittent burning, stabbing, or shooting pain perceived in the amputated part of the limb which occurs at rest and not necessarily with manipulation of the stump. This usually subsides with time, generally within 6 months. However, 10% of patients will experience chronic intractable phantom pain.[2] Pharmacological agents used for phantom pain are similar to those for neuropathic pain. These include amitriptyline, carbamazepine, and gabapentin.[3]

Wound Care and Oedema Control

Soft tissue swelling of the residual limb delays wound healing and causes pain. For a start, a soft dressing with an over-the-top elastic bandage wrapped in a figure-of-eight technique (Figure 1), compressive Tubigrip stockinet, or elastic shrinker is used. This is easily applied and allows for frequent wound inspection.

Contracture Prevention and Joint Range of Motion

As a result of the alteration of muscular balance and contraction of the wound after surgery, knee flexion contracture in transtibial amputees and

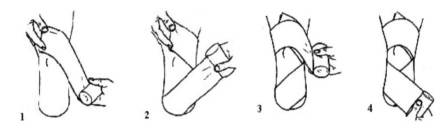

Figure 1:   Bandaging Technique for Below-knee Amputation

Notes:

1. Start with bandage held in place on inside of thigh just above knee and unroll bandage such that laid diagonally down outer side of stump while maintaining about two-thirds of maximum stretch in bandage.
2. Bring bandage over inner end of stump and diagonally up outer side of stump.
3. Bring bandage under back of knee, continue over upper part of kneecap and down under back of knee.
4. Bring bandage diagonally down back of stump and around over end of stump. Continue up back of stump to starting point on inside of thigh and repeat sequence in a manner such that entire stump is covered when roll is used up. It is important that tightest part of bandage be at end of stump.

Source: Adapted from Malaysian Information Network on Disabilities.

hip contracture in a flexed, abducted, and externally rotated position in transfemoral amputees occur.

A contracted joint affects the alignment of the limb when a prosthesis is applied and affects efficient ambulation. A knee flexion of more than 25 degrees and a hip abduction and flexion of more than 15 degrees in a below-knee amputee and above-knee amputee respectively will result in suboptimal prosthesis use.[4]

Prevention of contractures includes keeping the knee in an extended position at all times and the patient should sit with an extension board under the knee. The use of a pillow beneath the knee must be avoided.

A daily schedule for a range of motion and stretching exercises with counteracting muscle group strengthening exercises help prevent joint contracture (see NUH Rehabilitation Programme).

Physical Conditioning

Amputees need to learn new techniques of bed mobility and transfers to adapt to the change in their body mechanics. A pivot manoeuvre or use of a transfer board allows easy transfer from a bed to a chair. Detachable armrests on wheelchairs are recommended to accommodate these transfer skills.

Ambulation using walking frames for short distances is a targeted goal upon discharge. The training of balance using parallel bars is commenced in the early post-operative period (see NUH Rehabilitation Programme). The use of proper footwear and care for the contralateral limb must be emphasised. Patients with a cardiac disease history may require close monitoring during therapy sessions.

Psychological Support and Education

The prevalence of clinical depression and adjustment disorders is high in the early post-operative phase. Counselling is essential to reduce a patient's anxiety level and is more effective if practised at the pre-operative stage. This should include discussion of the necessity for amputation, rehabilitation process, estimated time of prosthesis fitting, and training with advice on projected functional outcome. Education on stump care and good glycaemic control are essential. Caregiver training may be required to assist with home management.

NUH Below-knee Rehabilitation Programme

Day 1

- Chest physiotherapy
- Straight leg raising (Figure 2)
- Hip abduction
- Isoquads (isometric/static quadriceps exercises) (Figure 3)
- Calf pumping (isometric gastrocnemius exercises)

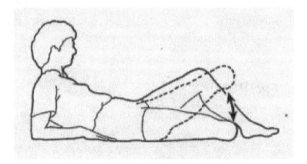

Figure 2:   Straight Leg Raising

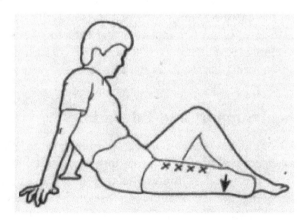

Figure 3:   Isoquads

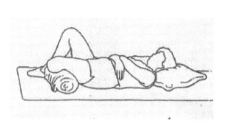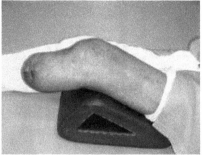

Figure 4: Stump Exercises

Day 2

- Thermoplastic splint fitting by occupational therapist.
- Inner range quadriceps or stump exercises (0–30 degrees knee flexion with roll of towel/support under thigh) (Figure 4).
- Standing with walking frame.
- Walking/balancing with walking frame.

Day 3

- Balancing across parallel bars at physiotherapy department orthopaedic gym.
- Surgical drain removed and outer dressings lightened.

Day 5

- Wound inspection (done earlier if dressing becomes soaked, foul odour is smelt, or patient develops a fever).
- Primapore dressing.
- Figure-of-eight technique stump bandaging three times a day.
- Tubigrip compressive stockinet or elastic shrinker (Figure 5) may be applied for wound.
- Oedema.
- Caregiver training on stump bandaging using 6 inches crepe bandage (on discharge patient must be prescribed two rolls of 6 inches crepe bandage).

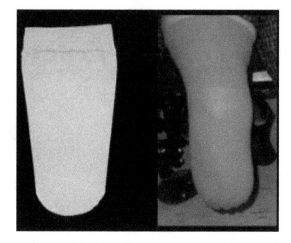

Figure 5:   Below-knee Elastic Stump Shrinker

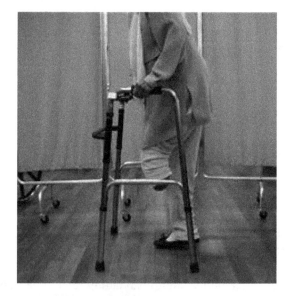

Figure 6:   Walking Frame Ambulation

Criteria for Discharge

Target: 1 week post-operatively

- Able to walk/balance with walking frame (Figure 6)
- Able to achieve stump control
- Caregiver proficiency with stump bandaging

Plan for Discharge

- Planning must begin on day patient was admitted for the diabetic foot problem by Case Manager and Nursing Officer in charge of ward.
- Caregiver training must be provided from the first post-op day.
- Lack of planning leads to unnecessary prolonged length of stay and increased hospitalisation cost.

Follow-Up Clinic Appointments

- **Orthopaedic Clinic:** Wound inspection and removal of sutures at 14th post-operative day or later (diabetics may take a longer time to heal — as long as 3 weeks or more).
- **Diabetic Clinic:** Diabetic control by endocrinologist and education on diabetes by nurse.
- **Podiatry:** Education on foot care for other leg and advice on footwear. +/– Cardiology, renal, ophthalmology clinic

Stump Preparation for Prosthesis Fitting

- Monthly serial measurement of stump girth during follow-up (Figure 7).
- Maximal stump shrinkage usually achieved after about 3–4 months.
- Prosthesis fitting at Artificial Limb Centre (in Singapore, there is a centralised prosthesis fitting centre for all hospitals in Tan Tock Seng Hospital, Figure 8).
- Commencement of rehabilitation walking exercises.

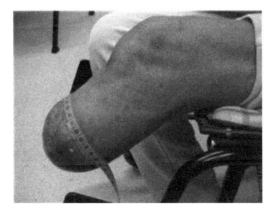

Figure 7: Stump Girth Measurement

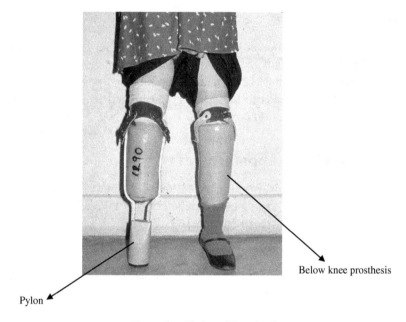

Below knee prosthesis

Pylon

Figure 8:   Fitting of Prosthesis

- Suitability of prosthesis checked after 2 weeks by prosthetist (in clinic at Tan Tock Seng Hospital) and Orthopaedic Surgeon in Diabetic Foot Clinic.

Cost of Prosthesis

The majority of our amputees belong to the lower socio-economic group. Many may not be able to afford purchasing the below-knee prosthesis. The cost of a prosthesis (subsidised by the Government) is about SGD $900. Those that cannot afford to buy the prosthesis must be referred to the Medico-Social Worker for financial assistance.

It is very encouraging to note that recently the Ministry of Health has given priority to diabetes mellitus to be one of the ten chronic diseases where health costs can be obtained from the patient's own Central Provident Fund. This has been a great help to our patients many of whom are poor.

References

1. H. Jung, Comprehensive post-operative management after lower limb amputations: current concepts in rehabilitation. *SGH Proc.* **16**: 58–62 (2007).
2. T.S. Jensen *et al.*, Immediate and long-term phantom limb pain in amputee: incidence, clinical characteristics and relationship to pre-amputation limb pain. *Pain.* **21**: 267–268 (1985).
3. M. Bone, P. Critchley, and D.J. Buggy, Gabapentin in postamputation phantom limb pain: a randomized, double-blind, placebo-controlled, cross-over study. *Reg Anesth Pain Med.* **27**: 481–486 (2002).
4. A. Moshirfar *et al.*, Prosthetic options for below knee amputation after osteomyelitis and nonunion of the tibia. *Clin Orthop.* **360**: 110–121 (1999).

Appendix A

NUH Diabetic Foot Team

Aziz Nather

Chairperson, Diabetic Foot Team, National University Hospital

Need for Diabetic Foot Service

In January 2003, Professor K. Satku, Chief of Orthopaedic Surgery, encouraged me to start a service for the diabetic foot. He was the Director of Medical Services in the Ministry of Health (MOH).

In May 2003, we formed a multidisciplinary foot team, involving an endocrinologist, an infectious disease specialist, a podiatrist, and nurses.

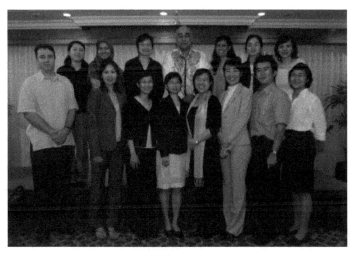

Pioneer NUH Diabetic Foot Team (November 2004)

309

NUH Diabetic Foot Team also designed a clinical pathway for the treatment of patients with diabetic foot problems. Its implementation was instrumental to the success of our foot team.

Together with the Diabetic Foot Clinical Pathway, the NUH multidisciplinary team for diabetic foot problems was launched in May 2003, with Dr. Nather as Chairperson and Dr. Chionh Siok Bee (Endocrinologist) as Co-Chairperson.

In each diabetic team round on Tuesday morning, cases were presented by the house officers in Ward 54. Each teaching round was awarded 1 point for Continuous Medical Education.

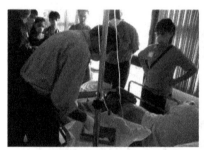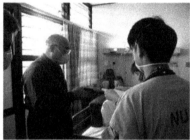

Patient Interaction and Wound Dressing During a Team Round

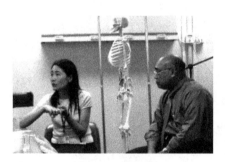

Explaining Clinical Pathway

The Diabetic Foot Clinical Pathway was finalised in January 2004. The pathway was carefully explained to each new batch of house officers by the Case Manager. All patients admitted to the ward were clerked using this pathway. In addition, we also ran a combined diabetic foot clinic on Wednesday mornings.

The results of our Team Approach and Clinical Pathway were presented during the keynote address delivered by Dr. Nather at the First

National and Regional Conference on Diabetic Foot Problems on 20 November 2004. This conference was attended by 220 participants (doctors, nurses, and allied health professionals) from Singapore, Malaysia, Indonesia, and Hong Kong.

The average length of stay decreased from 20.4 days (pre-team) to 13.7 days (post-team). The major amputation rate decreased significantly from 31.2% in 2002 to 19.6% in 2004. The complication rate was also reduced from 19.7% to 8.8%.

Research Teams for Diabetic Foot

Diabetic foot surgery offered good opportunities for research. Research teams comprising students who had just completed A-level education were formed. These were top students from Raffles Junior College, Hwa Chong Junior College, and Victoria Junior College who were keen to pursue medicine. They were attached from January to May.

First Research Team, 2005

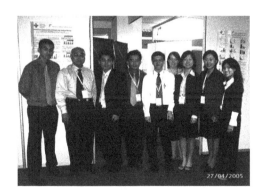 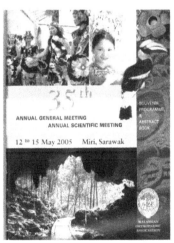

Zameer Aziz, Bernard Feng Min Chin, Clarabelle Lin Bitong, Christine Ong Hui Jing

- Predictive factors for limb loss
- Assessment of sensory neuropathy using neurometer
- Diabetic foot infections
- Diabetic footwear

Presented nine papers at 35th Malaysian Orthopaedic Association (MOA) Annual Conference in Miri, Sarawak in May 2005.

Second Research Team, 2006

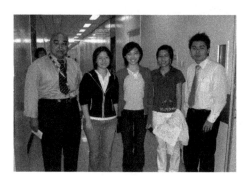 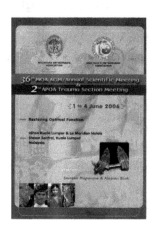

Alice Shu Hui Neo, Eileen Sim Yi Lin, Jocelyn Li Ling Chew

- Anodyne therapy for recalcitrant diabetic foot ulcers.
- Detecting neuropathy in early diabetics using neurometer assessment.

Presented five papers at the 36th MOA Annual Conference and 2nd APOA Trauma Section Meeting in Kuala Lumpur, Malaysia, in June 2006.

Third Research Team, 2007

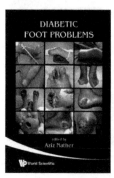 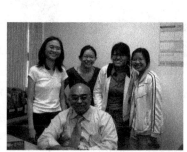 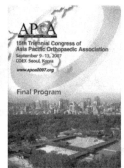

Janice Chien Chi Cheng, Li Xinyi, You Min Luah, Yan Limin

- Socio-economic profile of patients with diabetes foot complications

Presented five papers at the APOA 15th Triennial Congress in Seoul, Korea, in September 2007.

Assisted manuscript preparation for *Diabetic Foot Problems*, published by World Scientific in 2008.

Fourth Research Team, 2008

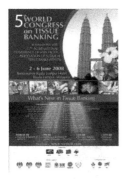
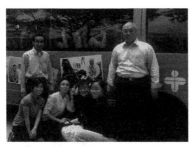
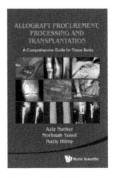

Low Jia Ming, Zheng Shushan, Pauline Chan Poh Lin, Vanessa Chang Chui Lian

- VAC dressings for diabetic wounds
- Outcomes of major and minor amputations

Presented two papers at the 38th Malaysian Orthopaedic Association (MOA) Annual Conference in Kuala Lumpur, Malaysia, in May 2008.

Assisted in manuscript preparation for *Allograft Procurement, Processing and Transplantation*, published by World Scientific in September 2010.

Fifth Research Team, 2009

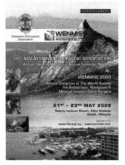
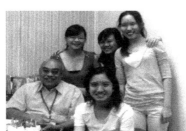
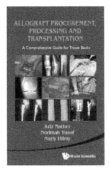

Audrey Han Yan Yi, Odelia Koh Si Qi, Patricia Tay Li Min, Valerie Chan Xin Bei

- VAC dressings for diabetic wounds
- Outcome of below-knee amputations

Presented four papers at the 39th MOA Annual Conference in May 2009 in Sabah, Malaysia.

Assisted manuscript preparation for *Allograft Procurement, Processing and Transplantation*, published by World Scientific in September 2010.

Sixth Research Team, 2010

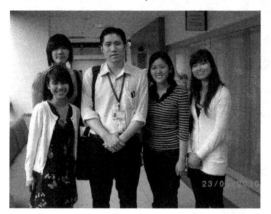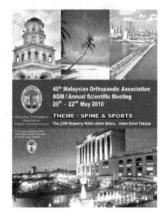

Loretta Wong Sue Mae, Jessica Ee Siqing, Jane Lim Su Juan, Kuang Silin

- The functional outcome of below-knee amputees and ray amputees with diabetic foot problems.
- The effect of Bridge VAC dressings.

Presented two papers at the 40th MOA Annual Conference in May 2010 held in Johor Bahru, Malaysia.

Seventh Research Team, 2011

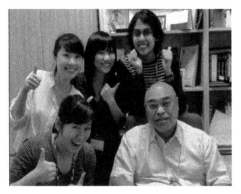 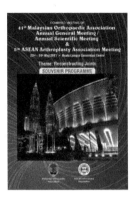

Chang Ziyuin, Tiffany Wong Tuck Chin, Ramiya Elangovan, Tessa Ong E-Lin

- The outcome of below-knee amputees and ray amputees with diabetic foot problems.
- Predictive factors for below-knee amputation in patients with diabetic foot problems (MOH Grant).

Presented two papers at the 41st MOA Annual Conference in May 2011 at KLCC in Kuala Lumpur, Malaysia.

Assisted in preparation of two papers for presentation at the 6th International Symposium on the Diabetic Foot in Noordwijkerhout in the Netherlands in May 2011.

Eighth Research Team, 2012

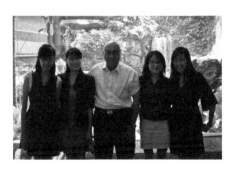 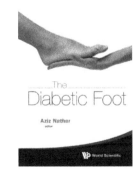

Amaris Lim Shu Min, Teo Zhen Ling, April Voon Siew Lian, Amy Pannapat Chanyarungrojn

- Predictive factors for below-knee amputations.
- Socio-economic factors in patients with diabetic foot problems.
- The role of oximeter in measuring tissue perfusion in diabetic foot patients.
- The oximeter as a measure of tissue perfusion in the normal foot.

Presented two papers at the 42nd MOA Annual Conference in June 2012 in Kuantan, Malaysia.

Assisted in manuscript preparation for *The Diabetic Foot*, published by World Scientific in September 2012.

Ninth Research Team, 2013

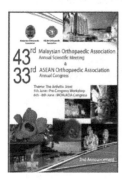
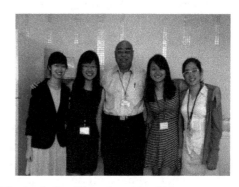

Elaine Tay Yiling, Jane Lim Jia Xin, Jamie Kee Xiang Lee, Mao Haitong

- Versajet hydrosurgery system
- Renasys-GO™ Negative Pressure Wound Therapy

Presented two papers at the 43rd MOA Annual Conference in May 2013 in Kuching, Sarawak.

Assisted in manuscript preparation for *Planning Your Research and How to Write It*, a guide for residents and young researchers embarking on research for the first time.

Tenth Research Team, 2014

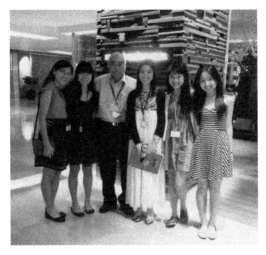

Claire Chan Shu-Yi, Wee Lin, Eda Lim Qiao Yan, Zest Ang Yi Yen, Joy Wong Ler Yi

Finalised and produced *Planning Your Research and How to Write It — A Comprehensive Guide for Young Researchers*, Aziz Nather (Editor, World Scientific), published in December 2015.

Eleventh Research Team, 2015

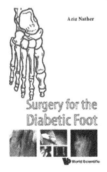
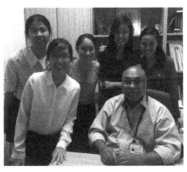

Rachel Teo Yi Lin, Ma Qian Hui, Julia Cheong Ling Yu, Tan Ting Fang, Amalina Anwar

Finalised and produced *Surgery for Diabetic Foot. An Operative Manual for Surgeons*, Aziz Nather (Editor, World Scientific), published in July 2016.

Started *Understanding Diabetic Foot — A Comprehensive Guide for General Practitioners*, Aziz Nather (Editor, World Scientific).

Twelfth Research Team, 2015

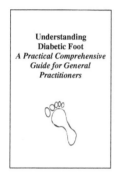

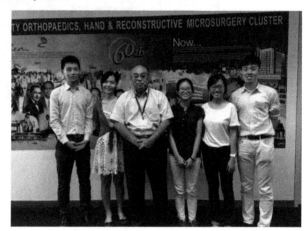

Cao Shuo, Jere Low Wenn, Sarah Lim Man Lin, Mae Chua Chui Wei, Danson Lim Kai Bing

Completed chapters for *Understanding Diabetic Foot — A Comprehensive Guide for General Practitioners*, Aziz Nather (Editor, World Scientific), in press, 2023.

Publications by NUH Diabetic Foot Team

Books

1. A. Nather (ed.), *Diabetic Foot Problems*, World Scientific (2008).
2. A. Nather (ed.), *The Diabetic Foot*, World Scientific (2013).
3. A. Nather (ed.), *Planning Your Research and How to Write It*, World Scientific (2015).
4. A. Nather (ed.), *Surgery For Diabetic Foot*, World Scientific (2016).

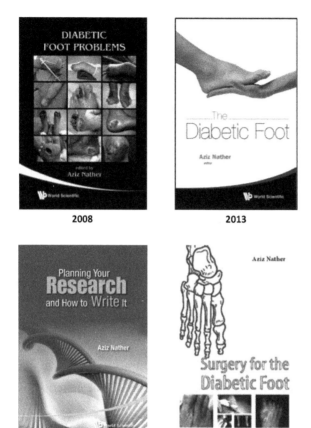

2008   2013

2015   2016

Book Chapter

A. Nather and F.C. Han, The diabetic foot, in: S. Sivananthan, E. Sherry, *et al.* (eds.), *Mercer's Textbook of Orthopaedics and Trauma,* Chapter 127, Hodder Education (2011).

Publications in Journals

1. A. Nather, S.B. Chionh, Y.H. Chan, J.L.L. Chew, C.B. Lin, S.H. Neo, and E.Y. Sim, Epidemiology of diabetic foot problems and predictive factors for limb loss, *J. Diabetes Complications.* **22**: 77–82 (2008).

2. A. Nather, S.H. Neo, S.B. Chionh, S.C.F. Liew, E.Y. Sim, and J.L.L. Chew, Assessment of sensory neuropathy in diabetic patients without diabetic foot problems, *J. Diabetes Complications.* **22**: 126–131 (2008).
3. A. Nather, S.B. Chionh, Y.Y. Han, P.L. Chan, and A. Nambiar, Effectiveness of vacuum-assisted closure (VAC) therapy in the healing of chronic diabetic foot ulcers, *Ann Acad Med Singapore.* **39**(5): 353–358 (2010).
4. A. Nather, S. B. Chionh, L. M. Tay, Z. Aziz, J. W. H. Teng, A. Nambiar, K. Rajeswari and A. Eramus, Foot screening for diabetics, *Ann Acad Med Singapore.* **39**(6): 472–474 (2010).
5. A. Nather, S.B. Chionh, K.L. Wong, S.Q.O. Koh, Y.H. Chan, X.Y. Li, and A. Nambiar, Socioeconomic profile of diabetic patients with and without foot problems, *Diabet Foot Ankle.* **1**: 5523–5531 (2010).
6. A. Nather, S.B. Chionh, K.L. Wong, X.B. Chan, L. Shen, P.A. Tambyah, A. Jorgensen, and A. Nambiar, Value of team approach combined with clinical pathway for diabetic foot problems: a clinical evaluation, *Diabet Foot Ankle.* **1**: 5731–5741 (2010).
7. A. Nather, Y.H. Ng, K.L. Wong, and J.A. Sakharam, Effectiveness of bridge VAC dressings in the treatment of diabetic foot ulcers, *Diabet Foot Ankle.* **2**: 5893–5900 (2011).
8. Z. Aziz, W.K. Lin, A. Nather, and C.Y. Huak, Predictive factors for lower extremity amputations in diabetic foot infections, *Diabet Foot Ankle.* **2**: 7463–7472 (2011).
9. A. Nather, K.L. Wong, Z. Aziz, C.H.J. Ong, B.M.C. Feng, and C.B. Lin, Assessment of sensory neuropathy in patients with diabetic foot problems, *Diabet Foot Ankle.* **2**: 6367–6377 (2011).
10. A. Nather, Short commentary (expert opinion) for "role of negative pressure wound therapy in healing", *J Surg Techniq Case Report.* **1**(1): 23–24 (2009).
11. A. Nather, and K.L. Wong, Distal amputations for the diabetic foot, *Diabet Foot Ankle.* **4**: 21288–21294 (2013).
12. K.L. Wong, A. Nather, L. Shen, Z. Cheng, T.C. Wong, and C.T. Lim, Clinical outcomes of below knee amputations in diabetic foot patients, *Ann Acad Med Singapore.* **42**: 388–394 (2013).
13. C.C. Hong, A. Nather, J.K.X. Lee, and H.T. Mao, Hydrosurgery is effective for debridement of diabetic foot patients, *Ann Acad Med Singapore.* **43**(8): 395–399 (2014).
14. K.L. Wong, A. Nather, A.P. Chanyarungrojn, L. Shen, T.E. Ong, R.D. Elangova, and C.T. Lim, Clinical outcomes of ray amputation in

diabetic foot patients, *Ann Acad Med Singapore.* **43**(8): 428–432 (2014).

15. R. Malhotra, C.S. Chan, and A. Nather, Osteomyelities in diabetic foot, *Diabet Foot Ankle.* **5**: 24445–24457 (2014).
16. A. Nather, K.L. Wong, A.S. Lim, Z.W.D. Ng, and H.W. Hey, The modified Pirogoff's amputation in treating diabetic foot infections: surgical technique and case report, *Diabet Foot Ankle.* **5** (2014).
17. S.Y.C. Chan, K.L. Wong, J.X.J. Lim, Y.L.E. Tay, and A. Nather, The role of Renasys-GO™ in the treatment of diabetic lower limb ulcers: a case series, *Diabet Foot Ankle.* **5**: 24718–24726 (2014).
18. C.C. Hong, K.J. Tan, A. Lahiri, and A. Nather, Use of a definitive cement spacer for simultaneous bony and soft tissue. Reconstruction of mid- and hindfoot diabetic neuroarthropathy: a case report, *J Foot Ankle Surg.* **54**(1): 120–125 (2015).
19. A. Nather, S. Soegondo, J.M.F. Adam, H.K.R. Nair, A.H. Zulkilfly, M.A.A. Villa, L.S. Tongson, S.Y.B. Chua, M. Wijeyaratne, N. Somasundaram, P. Mutirangura, and A. Chuangsuwanich, Best practice guidelines for ASEAN plus: management of diabetic foot wounds, *Sri Lanka J Diabetes Endocrinol Metabol.* **5**: 1–37 (2015).

Courses On Foot Screening

In May 2005, a National Health Group (NHG) task force for the diabetic foot was set up with two representatives from each hospital. The objective was to design and run a foot screening course for training nurses from three hospitals: NUH, TTSH, and AH. NHG provided a grant of $76,500. The project was led by Dr. Nather and Dr. Tay Jam Chin (Vascular Surgeon and Endocrinologist, TTSH) as Director and Co-Director, respectively.

The curriculum included education on foot care, footwear, and care for diabetes. The one-week course included hands-on examination for measurement of ABI, TBI, and neurothesiometer, in addition to a foot screening protocol. It ended with a theory and practical exam on foot screening for each nurse clinician.

First Training Course for Diabetic Foot Screening (2006)

The first NHG Training Course for Foot Screening was conducted in March 2006 with 11 students, including two occupational therapists from University Kebangsaan Malaysia (UKM).

Second Regional Training Course for Diabetic Foot Screening (2007)

The second Regional Training Course for Diabetic Foot Screening in March 2007 was subsequently organised by NUH with 28 nurse clinicians: 16 from Singapore, 10 from Malaysia, 1 from Indonesia, and 1 from Hong Kong.

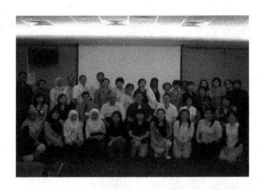

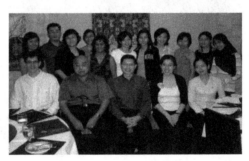

Third Regional Training Course for Diabetic Foot Screening (2008)

The third Regional Training Course for Diabetic Foot Screening followed in April 2008 with 43 participants: 29 from Singapore, 10 from Malaysia, 3 from Indonesia, and 1 from Hong Kong.

Fourth Regional Training Course for Diabetic Foot Screening (2010)

The fourth Regional Training Course continued in November 2010 with 20 participants: 12 from Singapore, 4 from Malaysia, 2 from Indonesia, and 2 from Hong Kong.

Fifth Regional Training Course for Diabetic Foot Screening (2011)

The fifth Regional Training Course for Diabetic Foot Screening was held from 21 to 25 November 2011. There were a total of 14 participants: 6 from Singapore, 7 from Malaysia, and 1 from Indonesia.

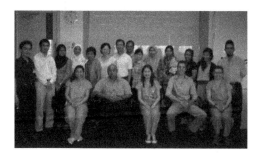

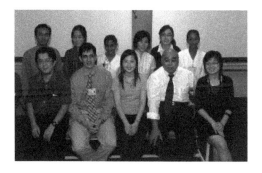

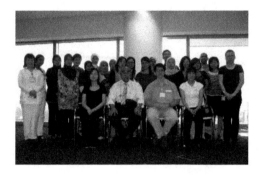

As of December 2011, a total of 116 nurse clinicians have been trained by the NUH foot screening courses, including 62 nurses from polyclinics and hospitals in Singapore, 31 nurses and 2 occupational therapists from Malaysia, 5 nurses and 2 orthopaedic surgeons from Indonesia, and 4 nurses from Hong Kong.

Conclusion

NUH employs a two-pronged strategy. The first strategy is prevention: providing annual foot screening for all diabetics to avoid the development of a diabetic foot complication. Once the complication develops, it is best treated by a diabetic foot team.

The NUH Diabetic Foot Team, together with the clinical pathway implemented, successfully decreased the major amputation rate in NUH from 31.2% (2002) to the present 11%. The team also plays an important role in promoting healthcare for diabetic foot patients in Singapore and the region.

Appendix B

History of Asia Pacific Association for Diabetic Limb Problems

Aziz Nather

Associate Professor, Honorary Secretary APADLP

Introduction

A regional association, the Asia Pacific Association for Diabetic Foot Problems, was formed in Singapore on 20 November 2004 during the first national and regional conference for diabetic foot problems held at the National University of Singapore from 20 to 21 November. 220 nurses and doctors from Malaysia, Indonesia, Hong Kong, and Singapore attended this conference. Dr. Nather was appointed Founding President, Dr. R. Ramanathan from Malaysia as President-Elect, Dr. Mulyono Soedirman from Indonesia as First Vice-President, and Dr. Josephine Ip from Hong Kong as Second Vice-President. The Guest-of-Honour was Dr. Balaji Sadasivan, Senior Minister of State for Health.

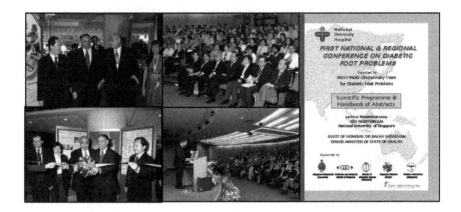

Subsequently, 11 conferences followed:

Second Asia Pacific Conference on Diabetic Foot Problems

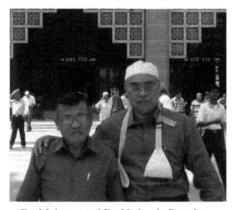

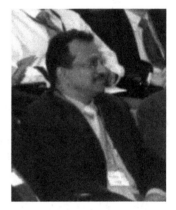

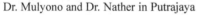

Dr. Mulyono and Dr. Nather in Putrajaya

- Organising Co-Chairpersons: Dr. R. Ramanathan and Dr. A. S. Naicker
- Venue: Putrajaya, Malaysia
- Date: 16–18 December 2005
- Number of participants: 200

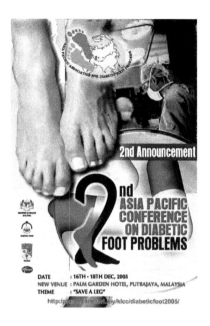
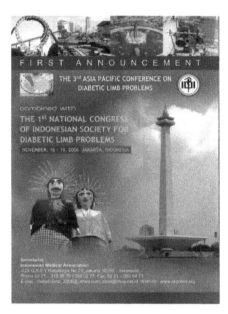

The association changed its name from APADFP to the Asia Pacific Association of Diabetic Limb Problems (APADLP). Diabetic problems included the upper limb (present in diabetics in 10% of cases).

Third APCDLP

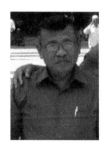

- Organising Chairperson: Dr. Mulyono Soedirman
- Venue: Ancor, Jakarta, Indonesia
- Date: 16–19 November 2006
- No. of participants: 200

Fourth APCDLP

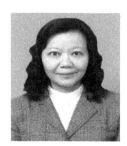
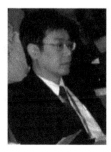

- Organising Co-Chairpersons: Dr. Josephine Ip Wing-Yuk and Dr. Joseph Wong Wing Cheung
- Venue: University of Hong Kong, Hong Kong
- Date: 23–25 November 2007

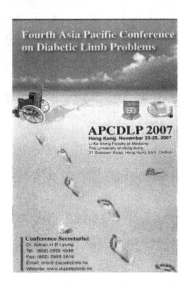

Fifth APCDLP

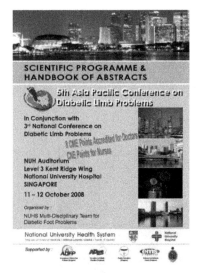

- Organising Chairperson: Dr. Aziz Nather
- Venue: National University Hospital, Singapore
- Date: 11–12 October 2008
- No. of participants: 250

The Guest-of-Honour was Professor K. Satku, Director of Medical Services. The team spent 2 years (2006–2007) writing *Diabetic Foot Problems*. It was launched during the Opening Ceremony of this conference.

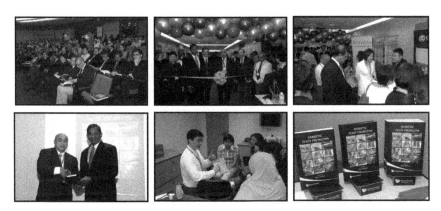

Sixth APCDLP

- Organising Chairperson: Dr. Xu Zhangrong
- Venue: Beijing, China

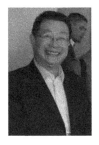

- Date: 14–16 August 2009
- No. of participants: 200

Guest lecturers included Dr. Benjamin Lipsky, Dr. David Armstrong, Dr. Andrew Boulton, and Dr. R.G. Frykberg.

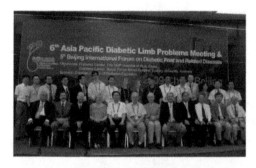

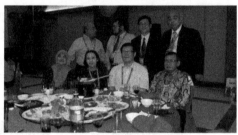

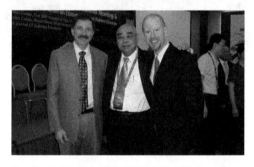

Benjamin Lipsky, Aziz Nather, David Armstrong

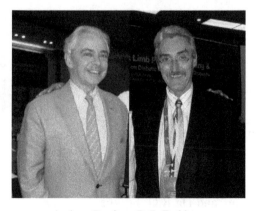

Andrew Boulton, R.G. Frykberg

Seventh APCDLP

- Organising Chairperson: Dr. Ahmad Hafiz Zulkifly
- Venue: Swissotel, Kuantan, Malaysia
- Date: 6–8 October 2010

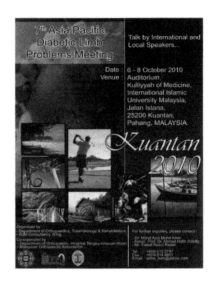

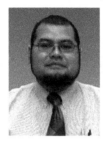

Eighth APCDLP

- Organising Chairperson: Dr. Bambang Tiksnadi
- Venue: Holiday Inn, Bandung, Indonesia
- Date: 16–17 November 2011

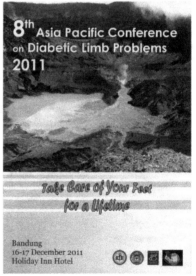

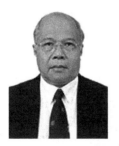

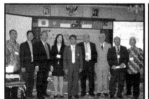
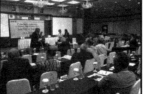
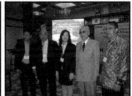

Ninth APCDLP

- Organising Chairperson: Dr. Samson Chan
- Venue: Mariner's Club, Hong Kong
- Date: 23–25 November 2011

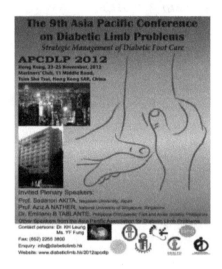

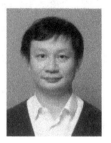

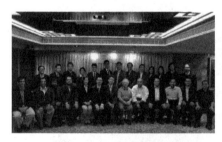

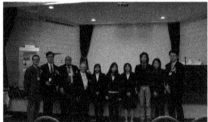

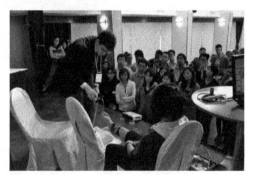

10th APCDLP

The 10th APCDLP, a landmark event in our Association's history, was held in the NUHS Auditorium in Singapore from 15 to 17 November 2013. 2013 was the 10th anniversary of APADLP as well as of the NUH Diabetic Foot Team.

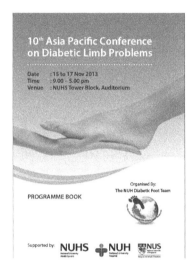

For this gala event, a one-day Nursing Certificate Course on Management of Diabetic Foot Wounds for nurses was organised on 15 November followed by the main conference. Guest speakers included 16 regional and 27 local experts. The scientific programme included 6 plenary lectures and 6 symposia. Novel events included a "Young Investigator Award" and a "Poster Paper Award".

The conference included a Trade Exhibition with 6 exhibition booths and 8 table displays.

There were 3 Gold Sponsors: Smith & Nephew, KCI, and Convatec.

A special 10th Anniversary Celebration Dinner was held on 16th November at The Glass House, Fort Canning Hotel in Fort Canning Park.

A special 10th Anniversary Commemorative Programme Handbook was also published with Claire Chan as the editor.

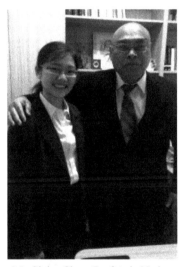

Ms Claire Chan, Prof Aziz Nather

11th APCDLP

- Organising Chairman: Dr. Geoff Sussman
- Venue: Monash University — Parkville Campus, VIC, Australia
- Date: 14–15 November 2014

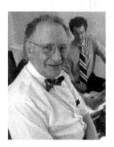

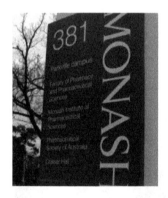

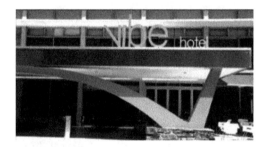

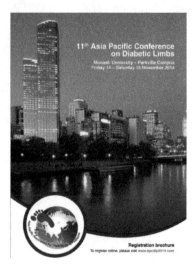

12th APCDLP

- Organising Chairman: Dr. Ahmad Hafiz Zulkifly
- Venue: Crescent IIUM, Kuala Lumpur, Malaysia
- Date: 5–6 November 2015

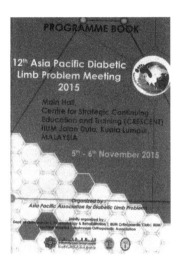

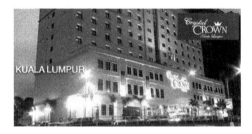

13th APCDLP

- Organising Chairman: Dr. Bambang Tiksnadi
- Venue: Jogjakarta, Indonesia
- Date: 8–9 October 2016

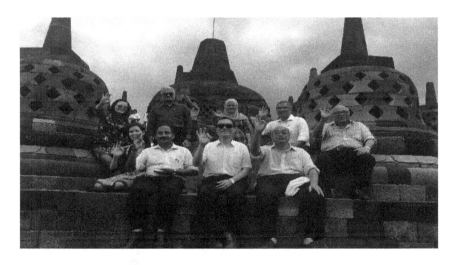

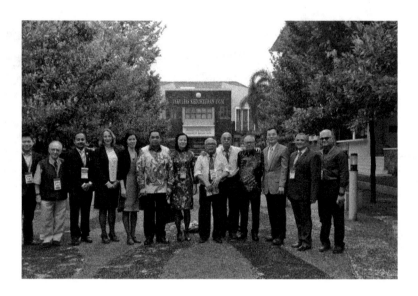

14th APCDLP

- Organising Chairmen: Dr. Apirag Chuangsuwanich and Ms. Gulapar Srisawasdi
- Venue: Faculty of Medicine, Siriraj Hospital.
  Mahidol University.Bangkok, Thailand
- Date: 17–19 November 201

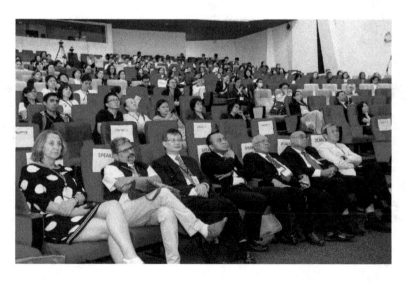

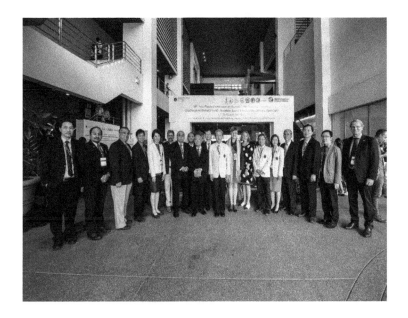

15th APCDLP

- Organising Chairman: Dr. Yur-ren Kuo
- Venue: Kaohsiung Medical University Hospital
  Kaohsiung, Taiwan
  Date: 26–28 October 2018

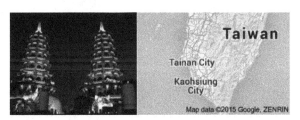

Kaohsiung

Municipality in Taiwan

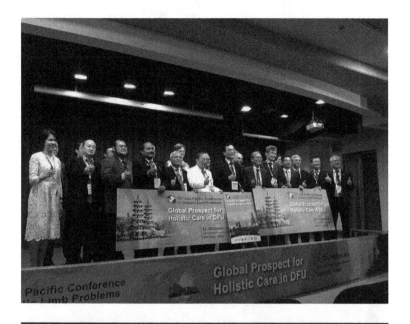

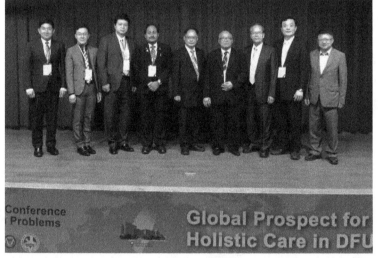

16th APCDLP

- Organising Chairman: Dr. Harikrishna R. Nair
- Venue: Berjaya Times Square Hotel
  Kuala Lumpur, Malaysia
- Date: 18–20 October 2019

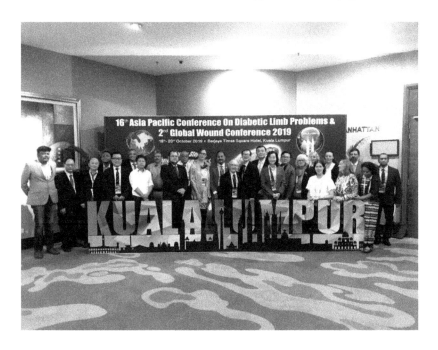

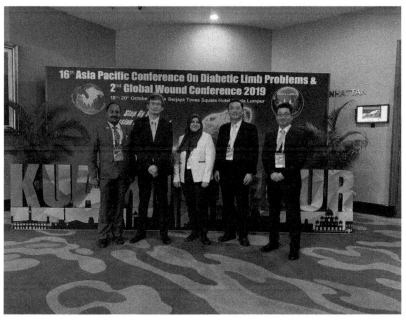

17th APCDLP

- Organising Chairmen: Dr. Eleanor Letran, Dr. Luinio S. Tongson, and Dr. Emiliano B. Tablante
- Venue: Manila, Philippines
- Date: 16–18 June 2021

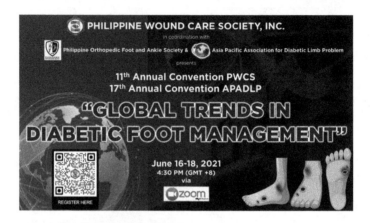

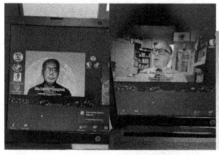
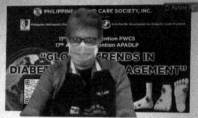

Next Three Conferences

- **18th Conference**
  Goa, India
  14–16 October 2022
- **19th Conference**
  Melbourne, Australia
  October/November 2023

- **20th Conference**
  Singapore
  October/November 2024
  20th Anniversary of APADLP

Office Bearers of APADLP from 2000 to 2002

President	Harikrishna K.R. Nair	Malaysia
President Elect	Gulapar Srisawasdi	Thailand
First Vice President	Yur-Ren Kuo	Taiwan
Second Vice President	Nicoletta Frescos	Australia
Honorary Secretary	Aziz Nather	Singapore
Assistant Hon Secretary	Chee Yu Han	Singapore
Honorary Treasurer	Gillian Butcher	Australia
Auditors	Geoff Sussman	Australia
	Josephine Ip Wing-Yuk	Hong Kong

Past Presidents of APADLP

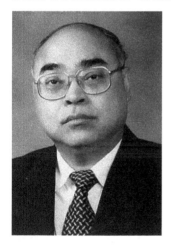

Aziz Nather
Singapore
Founding President
2004–2006

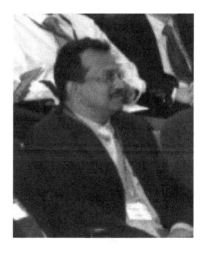

R. Ramanathan
Ipoh, Malaysia
2nd President
2006–2008

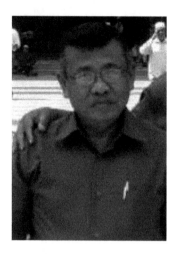

Mulyono Soedirman
Jakarta, Indonesia
3rd President
2008–2010

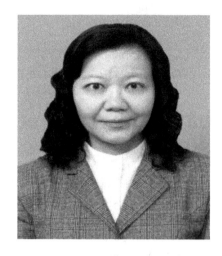

Josephine Ip Wing-Yuk
Hong Kong
4th President
2010–2012

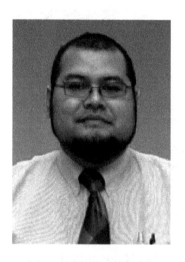

Ahmad Hafiz Zulkifly
Kuantan, Malaysia
5th President
2012–2014

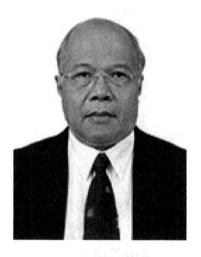

Bambang Tiksnadi
Bandung, Indonesia
6th President
2014–2016

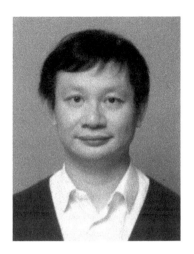

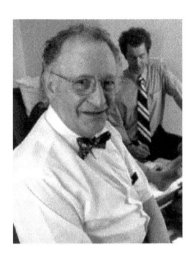

Samson Chan Chi Fa
Hong Kong
7th President
2016–2018

Geoffrey Sussman
Melbourne, Australia
8th President
2018–2021